How to cope with almost anything with hypnotherapy

DANIEL FRYER

How to cope with almost anything with hypnotherapy

Simple ideas to enhance your wellbeing and resilience

GREEN TREE
LONDON · OXFORD · NEW YORK · NEW DELHI · SYDNEY

GREEN TREE
GREEN TREE Bloomsbury Publishing Plc
50 Bedford Square, London, WC1B 3DP, UK
29 Earlsfort Terrace, Dublin 2, Ireland

BLOOMSBURY, GREEN TREE and the Green Tree logo are trademarks of
Bloomsbury Publishing Plc

First published in Great Britain 2024

A catalogue record for this book is available from the British Library.

Library of Congress Cataloguing-in-Publication data has been applied for.

ISBN: TPB: 978-1-3994-1117-2; eBook: 978-1-3994-1118-9;
ePdf: 978-1-3994-1116-5

2 4 6 8 10 9 7 5 3 1

Text design and illustrations by Austin Taylor
Typeset in IBM Plex Serif by Deanta Global Publishing Services, Chennai, India
Printed and bound in Great Britain by CPI Group (UK) Ltd., Croydon, CR0 4YY

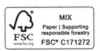

To find out more about our authors and books visit www.bloomsbury.com and
sign up for our newsletters.

Note: The information provided in this book is not intended to be a substitute for
professional advice or consultation with a health professional.

Client examples are from real therapy sessions, but their names have been
changed to protect individual privacy.

For Lara
Gone, but never, ever forgotten.

Contents

HYPNOTHERAPY RECORDINGS

QR CODE

Scan the QR code below for accompanying audio clips.

Scan me!

Credit: Freepik

This QR code will take you to a website to access the hypnotherapy recordings.

https://www.bloomsbury.com/hypnotherapyaudio

Look out for this symbol throughout the book and return to this page to scan the above QR code.

If you have any difficulties accessing this page, contact greentree@bloomsbury.com.

Prologue

You will discover later in this book exactly why someone who says they can't be hypnotised can't be hypnotised. But if you make it to the end of this prologue, you will have had a little taste of hypnosis (a trance-like state very similar to daydreaming). You will have also discovered that not everyone who wants to be successfully hypnotised for something will be successfully hypnotised for something. Hypnotherapy works best when the suggestions are positive (something that you do want rather than something that you don't want) and, for certain things, such as breaking bad habits, success will depend to a large degree on just how much you want to give up that thing you say you want to give up and, to a lesser degree, on just how much you like, trust or have confidence in your chosen hypnotherapist. Science says you form your first impression of someone within the first seven seconds of meeting them. It also suggests that our first impressions are incredibly accurate. I must be doing something right because, as far as I know, my success rate is pretty good. Even if your first impression of hypnosis is not.

Inéz came to see me for help with stopping smoking having already been to see another hypnotherapist for the same thing just a few months before. Sadly, hypnotherapy hadn't worked, and she had had a cigarette the very next day. When I asked her why she thought that might be, she admitted two things. First, that she hadn't been that committed to quitting at the time (but having reflected on things since, now thought that she was) and, second, she hadn't really liked the hypnotherapist's voice.

'I found it rather grating,' she said. This isn't a good quality to possess if you want to lull people into an altered state of consciousness and be there to provide therapeutic suggestions in calm and inviting tones.*

I took a full case history from Inéz, including every single aspect of her smoking habit, from the very first one of the morning to the very last one of the night, noting any variations over the course of the week. I also took note of her specific triggers (such as stress, and people, and places and so on), found out what she thought hypnotherapy was and how it was supposed to work, and highlighted what she could reasonably expect to experience from hypnosis (correcting any misconceptions she may have picked up along the way). In addition, I asked her what the main benefits to quitting for her were.

A big one was her house. It was yellowed by tobacco smoke, it felt grimy, the air was redolent but stale and, although her non-smoking friends could pick up on the lingering tobacco tang more than she could, she still found it rather unpleasant. She hated what her habit had done to her home. I asked her what she would like her environment to smell of when she no longer smoked, once it was fresh and clean and her senses had improved.

'Lavender,' she said. 'I love the smell of lavender.' She lived in a downstairs flat, with a small garden and a set of French windows in the living room leading out to that garden, which contained three or four rather large lavender bushes of different varieties (including English and French). It also contained honeysuckle, a few roses, an apple tree and a herb garden. On a nice day, Inéz would open the windows and the breeze would gently waft the relaxing aroma of lavender, the sweet scent of honeysuckle and, sometimes, even the enticing bouquets of mint and rosemary – two plants to which lavender is related – into her living room. Inéz's friends who did not smoke would always find the fragrances far more tantalising than she did, and she longed to experience them at the same intensity.

And so, I helped Inéz drift into a hypnotic trance, making my voice sound extra warm and sultry as I did so and then, once her trance was deep enough for the work to begin, not only did I break her smoking habit cigarette by cigarette, but I also gilded the proverbial lily by heavily evoking the sights, scents and experience of both the lavender and the

---

* This doesn't mean that the therapist had a grating voice, only that Inéz found it grating. Them's the breaks.

honeysuckle, as well as the various herbs and other flowers and bushes in her garden. I talked of warm summer breezes; I waxed lyrical about the gentle drone of the many honey bees and bumblebees that were attracted by the colours and nectars of the various flowers; I mentioned apple tree leaves rustling in the wind; I described birdsong, and I painted the various purple and mauve hues of the different varieties of lavender as I brought to mind the gentle, calming aromas combining and wafting into her beautiful, clean, crisp living room as she relaxed in her favourite chair on a beautiful day. I even remained silent for a few minutes to let her enjoy the panorama her mind had created around my suggestions for a little while longer. Eventually, I ended the session and brought her back to full waking consciousness.

A smile widened from ear to ear as she stretched out and opened her eyes. 'Mm, lavender,' she said. 'I can smell it. It's so lovely.'

Four weeks later, she sent me an email saying she hadn't smoked a single cigarette since her session with me, had redecorated the living room and – with a newfound sense of olfactory joy – was already appreciating all the fragrances wafting in through her open French windows.

Now, if you have not only read the above paragraphs, but have found yourself immersed in them, if your surroundings faded away and you were transported to a lavender-filled garden, even if just for a moment; if you could almost see yourself wandering around it and admiring the beautiful flowers and shrubs; if you could almost see the flowers gently swaying in the breeze, or almost heard the drone of the bees; if you, like Inéz, could almost smell the lavender then you have just experienced a state of trance very similar to hypnosis, right now, as you read this book. Wherever you are reading this passage – at home, in a coffee shop or in a bookstore – as you lost yourself in the words on this page, you drifted into a trance-like state.

Hypnosis is easy and natural; we drift in and out of these altered states of consciousness several times a day, often without even realising it but, as you get to grips with this book, you are going to get very good at it and you are going to do some amazing things with it. If you put the practice in, you are most definitely going to enhance your wellbeing, increase your resilience and give yourself a newfound sense of peace and harmony.

If you would like to know more about why this is, if you have enjoyed this little experience of hypnosis and are keen to know more, if you really would like to feel calmer and more in control in a world that feels increasingly out of kilter, then please read on. Hypnotherapy really can help you cope with almost anything and, if you've made it this far, chances are you already trust me when I say that this is so.

In the next chapter, I shall be talking about what, exactly, it is that this book can help you cope with. But first – and, literally, as your first taste of the power of suggestion – I want you to imagine that you are sucking on a slice of lemon. No, really, I do.

Sucking on a lemon

Your imagination is very powerful. It is also suggestible. Under the right set of circumstances that is. This is how hypnotherapy works.

In a few minutes, I'm going to ask you to close your eyes. And, when I do, I want you to imagine that you are sucking on a fresh but sour, bitter, tangy and juicy slice of lemon. Maybe you are chopping one up for culinary purposes, ready to squeeze the juice out and add to a recipe. Perhaps you are making a cake or a curd. Maybe that juice has dribbled all over your hands and fingers and you are popping those fingers into your mouth to lick them clean. Maybe you've got a nice slice of lemon floating in a large, clear glass of your favourite brand of gin and fizzing tonic water. Perhaps it is drifting around in a glass of something a little more sober and refreshing, such as soda water and lime cordial. Are there any ice cubes in these drinks? Are they clinking musically against the sides of their respective glass tumblers? Either way, you have fished that slice of lemon out and popped it into your mouth. And you are now rolling that slice of lemon all around your mouth, letting its juice flow all over your tongue. Every drop of that fresh but sour, bitter, tangy and juicy lemon is tantalising your tastebuds. Once you have responded to the imaginary taste of that lemon – or appreciated it for as long as you wished to appreciate it – you can then open your eyes.

Read the above paragraph again if you need to and then, when you are ready, close your eyes and really allow yourself to see and sense and imagine sucking on that fresh but sour, bitter, tangy and juicy slice of lemon. Take as long as you wish.

Now that you have opened your eyes, I want you to think about your response. Did your mouth contract, or pucker, or water at the thought of that lemon? Did you salivate, did your mouth go a little dry, did you gulp or swallow? Chances are, you did. Which means your body responded, not to the taste of lemon but to the *suggestion* of the taste of lemon. The power of suggestion and the power of our imagination to act upon these suggestions is very important in hypnotherapy. Now, let's talk about what that can help you with.

PART ONE

AN OVERVIEW OF HYPNOSIS, HYPNOTHERAPY AND THE MIND

What this book is for

Are you exhausted? I know I am. Do you often feel like you're at the end of your tether and that it is about to break? Me too. And I'm a therapist. Not only that, but I practise self-hypnosis on a regular basis and meditate twice a day.

This is a book that is not only about hypnotherapy but also all the wonderful things you can do with it. Hypnotherapy can help enhance you both physically and mentally and, in turn, help you cope with just about anything life throws at you.

Life has always been stressful but lately it's been extra-stressful, what with the pandemic and other major events. If it's not one thing, then it's another and, if it's not that, then (as more than one client of mine has put it), 'it's everything all at once.'*

The seemingly never-ending series of crises and calamities have pushed most of us to the feathered edges of our coping strategies, taxed our nervous systems to their very limits (more on that later) and thrust one subject to the top of the personal and professional agenda. And that topic is 'wellbeing'.

---

* There is a hypnotherapy script I wrote myself years and years ago as a pick-me-up (after coughs, colds and flu etc.). I've included it in Chapter 8 on Stress and How to Handle It (*see* pp. 82–84). It's helped me on many an occasion (and continues to do so). I hope it does the same for you.

People are honouring it, treasuring it and working on it like never before. People are quite happy to ditch their jobs if they feel that their wellbeing is not being looked after or, worse, infringed upon.

One of the most important things many prospective employees want to know of any potential new employer is what their wellbeing policy looks like. In a massive job interview about-face, it's sometimes the interviewee who is leading the interview, with 'What is your wellbeing policy?' being a commonly asked question.

Hot on the heels of that topic is the subject of resilience, as one enhances the other and vice versa. I deliver a lot of workplace wellness webinars and live presentations to a variety of corporate clients, all trying to safeguard their employees' wellbeing and enhance their resilience in the face of stress. However, the best person to safeguard and enhance those things is you. But to look after them, you need to know what they are.

Also known as wellness, wellbeing refers to someone's value or quality of life. It can be summed up with an often-asked therapy question, 'Are you surviving or thriving?' This simple question can always elicit valuable information, regularly reveals a wide variety of responses and can, quite often, bring about floods of tears (mostly cathartic, thankfully).

More important than the concept of wellbeing is the idea of 'subjective' wellbeing. How do you rate, report and experience your life? Are you happy? Are you satisfied? Do you feel calm and in control of your life and its attendant circumstances, or do you feel like you're losing the plot?

Because of everything that has happened over the past few years, namely the pandemic, more people are reporting the latter as opposed to the former. Which is why people are leaving jobs not only because they don't support them but also because they're re-evaluating their lives and, with it, their sense of self.

Resilience, meanwhile, refers to our ability to adapt to change, deal with difficult circumstances and bounce back from challenge. It's a measure of how quickly we recover from a challenging event or situation.

Human beings are turning to all sorts of tools to help themselves feel happier, saner, more sorted and more balanced in this often out-of-kilter world. Mental health issues have soared. Chronic stress is rife. There is an edge. Some people have gone over it already. Many others are approaching it a lot faster than they would like. People are not only seeking out therapists in droves but discovering or rediscovering all sorts of physical and mental practices to enhance and energise their lives, to recharge both body and mind.

And they are returning to hypnotherapy.

Hypnotherapy and hypnosis are two different things. You will find that out as you delve deeper into this book. Hypnotherapy, in one form or another, has been around for centuries. It is one of the oldest forms of healing known to humans and has fallen out of favour more than once or twice.

That said, because what goes around does indeed come around (not just with karma but also with business), the media and the wellbeing industry are touting hypnotherapy as the next big wellness trend. At the time of writing, and according to the latest research, the hypnotherapy market is going to experience significant growth until at least 2030. One broadsheet newspaper reported that people on lengthy NHS waiting lists for psychotherapy were turning to hypnotherapy as a stopgap. Some were even eschewing one in favour of the other. Spas and resorts are using it to bolster their wellness offerings and hypnotherapists around the globe are all reporting a massive uptake in enquiries.

Hypnotherapy, then, is most definitely back on the menu.

However, I'm not just a hypnotherapist. I'm also a practitioner of rational emotive behaviour therapy (REBT), which is a form of cognitive behavioural therapy (CBT). I also like to make good use of tools and techniques from positive psychology. As I explain later, both REBT and positive psychology dovetail rather neatly with hypnotherapy. Together, there is a lot you can do with them.

For most of my therapeutic career, I've worked with anxiety disorders and work-related stress management (and still do). However, an increasing number of referrals are from people asking if I can just help them feel happier, calmer and more energised or give them strategies to cope. When I ask them what they want to feel happier with, or calmer in the face of, or what they want more energy or those coping strategies for, their usual response is, 'everything'.

I always say I can, of course, and I help them with hypnotherapy, REBT and positive psychology. To do this, I use many of the tools, tips and hypnotherapy scripts you are going to find in this book.

I have also used hypnotherapy, as well as REBT and positive psychology, to help me navigate my own life's ups and downs (of which there have been many). I've used them to mitigate stress, boost my coping strategies in the face of incredibly difficult life events and help me deal with whatever life has flung at me (health problems, relationship break-ups, interpersonal difficulties, redundancy, you name it) to the best of my abilities.

Over the years, I've helped hundreds of people to do the same. And I'd like to help you, too.

How this book is built

The topics in this book reflect many of the issues that my one-to-one clients bring me, as well as the goals they would like to achieve, but also the issues I have faced. With each topic, there is an overview, a case history or two, some stories from both a personal and professional level, a 'script' for you to use (if you decide to use self-hypnosis) and a recording to play (if you don't), which you can access online.

Part One of this book is all about the set-up. This is important as, without it, people rarely experience the full benefits of hypnotherapy. With that in mind, I spend a good amount of time setting things up well in the first face-to-face hypnotherapy session I have with someone, and I am also going to do it with you in this section. Here, you will find out how and why you can trust me to deliver hypnotherapy safely and expertly; you'll be given an overview of hypnosis and hypnotherapy (which has a very interesting and varied history); and will learn about the crucial differences and occasional similarities between stage hypnosis and hypnotherapy. I'll also be teaching you self-hypnosis and discussing a few other things that will help you along the way (including how to become good at anything, the brain and neuroplasticity, how to build a habit and how to stick to a goal). These are very reassuring to know before you go into a hypnotic trance. They're also good things to be reading while you practise your self-hypnosis, in advance of doing any therapy with it, as you need to be reasonably good at it before you apply any therapy suggestions.

If you don't like the idea of self-hypnosis, then many of the hypnotherapy exercises in this book are available to listen to straight to your smartphone or tablet using a modern, funky QR code.* The following code will take you to a dedicated page with a playlist of the recordings; you can also find this on page 8 while you are working through the book. Look out for this symbol ◀)) for a handy reminder that you can access recordings online.

---

* First invented in 1994 for the automotive industry in Japan, QR codes can today track products, manage documents, arrange redeliveries, check lottery tickets and now, download my voice straight into your brain via your music app (only for the purposes of good, I hasten to add).

Part Two of this book is all about enhancing various aspects of your wellbeing, including some of the most common issues I work on with clients: how to mitigate stress, stop negative thinking, focus on the positive, break bad habits, deal with insomnia, and more.

Part Three is where you'll be building your resilience. Here, you will learn how to cope with all the things you think you cannot cope with (including uncertainty, a lack of control over your life and constant change). As part of this, you will not only learn a whole lot more about REBT, but also discover how to become more assertive.

Traditional hypnotherapy is considered eclectic, in that a hypnotherapist is free to borrow from any therapy, any discipline and any school of thought, and use them in a variety of ways, or in the best way they think will help their client achieve whatever it is they want to achieve. I'll be borrowing mainly, but not exclusively, from REBT and positive psychology (and will be explaining what these therapies are, and how they can help you, along the way).

Before you carry on reading, however, I just want to address one thing. If you are suffering from a chronic condition or have an acute mental health diagnosis, then alongside this book, I would strongly recommend that you seek out the services of a professional.

Also, there are a few caveats regarding hypnotherapy. Most people can go into a trance to some degree or other. Some can't. First up, there are those who simply don't believe it will work. If you are one of those people, then you're correct and hypnotherapy can't help you. You will find out why later (*see* p. 36). However, if you've read this far, chances are, you're not one of those people. Also, if you are suffering from schizophrenia or have been diagnosed with panic disorder, it's best that you don't use hypnotherapy without a trained professional. And, if you are addicted to anything serious (recreational drugs, pharmaceutical drugs or alcohol) and are using regularly and/or heavily, hypnosis won't work until you've been clean and dry for a good few months. Doughnuts are fine. Also, if you are on a lot of medication, or medication for severe psychiatric illnesses, it's best you consult your doctor before attempting any form of hypnotherapy.

So, chronic or acute conditions (and hypnotherapy exclusions) aside, if you would like to improve your wellbeing and enhance your resilience, then please read on.

I've been successfully helping people deal with their problems and achieve their goals using either/or hypnotherapy, REBT and positive psychology since 2004 and I still often marvel at all its wonderous effects and outcomes.

The weird thing is, as you will discover in the next chapter, I never intended to be a therapist of any kind at all.

Why me?

Until just before my mid-30s, all my studies and most of my working life had centred around the media. My college studies involved it. My first degree was in journalism, and that was the industry I was working in.

At that point, my only understanding of hypnosis was by way of entertainment, mainly because I had been shot dead in front of a baying mob by a bloke with an egg whisk. That sort of thing tends to stay with you for a while.

I was shot by a stage hypnotist

I was 27 and studying at university. A stage hypnotist was brought in for a boozy entertainment night at the student union. One young man – a big, burly member of the rugby team – volunteered to be part of the act and came up on stage. He was hypnotised into thinking he was Arnold Schwarzenegger as The Terminator, given a rotary eggbeater, and told to go out into the crowd and then locate and terminate the first bald, bearded man he found. There was only one bald, bearded man in the crowd that night and he was me. I later found out that my mates had slipped the stage hypnotist a tenner before his act to make me part of his routine. The burly chap descended the stage and walked stiffly and robotically through the crowd of students, head and eyes scanning from left to right until he found me, zeroed in on my location, marched over to where I was and then, without a second's hesitation, terminated me with his spinning egg whisk. I pretended to die with dramatic effect. My friends still have the photos to prove it.

The altered state of consciousness that my Terminator guy was in was a hypnotic trance, but what the entertainer did with trance and what hypnotherapists do with trance are two very different things.

Hypnotherapy fell from favour when hypnosis became a form of vaudevillian entertainment back in the Victorian era. It still gets tarred with that brush even today. However, on the plus side, hypnotherapy is recognised by both the British Medical Association (BMA) and the National Institute for Health and Care Excellence (NICE). The BMA is the professional body and trade union for doctors in the UK, while NICE is part of the Department of Health in England. Hypnotherapy is also recognised and used by the NHS. The National Hypnotherapy Society is even an accredited registrant with the Professional Standards Authority (PSA), which puts it right up there with the British Association for Counselling and Psychotherapy (BACP) and the UK Council for Psychotherapy (UKCP). And, because of the amount of research that now exists, hypnotherapy is considered by many to be an evidence-based practice.

The thing with hypnotherapy is that it is never what you think it is. It very rarely feels like you think it's going to feel, and you rarely experience what you think you are going to experience. In fact, following their first hypnotherapy session, most people don't even think they've been hypnotised. I certainly didn't.

Close your eyes and relax...

I was about to write a feature. The idea was to collect a large group of people who wanted to give up smoking and get them to try various ways and means. This was for a health magazine for a pharmacy chain, and we were going to focus mainly on the nicotine replacement therapies (NRTs). One person was going to quit using gum, while another was going to try patches and so on. However, they also wanted to include other methods, including the original *Allen Carr's Easy Way to Stop Smoking* book, acupuncture and hypnotherapy. The idea was to interview all the quitters at the start of the journey and then again, regularly, at three-month intervals over the course of a year to see who stayed the course and who fell by the wayside.

At that time, I smoked (about ten on a good day, but way more if I went out and got drunk). I wanted to quit, liked the sound of the hypnotherapist I had talked to over the phone, put myself forward as the subject for that method, and took myself off to a very reputable hypnotherapist in Harley Street.*

You'd be forgiven for thinking, at this point in the book, that hypnotherapy is only good for stopping smoking. It's not but, like Inéz in the Prologue, I was introduced to hypnotherapy at a time when stopping smoking was in the hearts and minds of a great many people. And, let's face it, if you can stop someone from smoking, what can't you do with it?

I remember the session vividly. I sat in a comfy chair in a nice but innocently bland therapy room done out in shades of beige and magnolia. It was set quite far back in a ramshackle building that looked more like a house than a therapy practice. My hypnotherapist was male, grey of hair, warm of voice and comfortable of clothing.

As I did a few years later with Inéz, my hypnotherapist elicited a very detailed picture of my smoking habit and then thoroughly explained hypnosis and hypnotherapy to me, before answering any questions that I had and addressing any concerns, such as 'Will it work?', 'Can I be hypnotised?' and 'Will I say anything I will regret during the session?' (Yes, yes and no).

When I had no more questions or concerns, the hypnotherapy session began. Using the sound of his voice, he helped lull me into an altered state of consciousness and, when he thought my trance was at a deep enough level, broke my smoking habit.

I thought it was a load of old rubbish, to be honest. I did not feel hypnotised, and I was able to recall every single word he had said. I sat in that comfy chair, with my eyes closed, for a good 45 minutes or more and, all the way through the hypnotherapy session, I kept thinking, 'I can open my eyes any time I want. I can. Any time I want. I can. Any. Time. I know I can.' But I didn't. Not until the therapist asked me to. I thought I was just being polite.

It was raining when I left his clinic. Normally, I hate the rain but not this time. Everything about London in the wet looked extra sparkly and shiny as I walked down the street. The droplets of water had never looked so beautiful, and the way they reflected the light had never looked so absorbing. The reds and yellows and greens of the traffic lights along the

---

* Not that the location makes you reputable. Anyone can practise there. You can graduate (or not) and set yourself up as a 'Harley Street therapist' the very next day if there is a room available and you can afford the rent.

way had never looked so red or yellow or green. I felt very happy, euphoric even, but also very calm and serene.*

But at this point, I still didn't think I'd been hypnotised.

Stupidly, I'd arranged to meet a bunch of mates down the pub immediately after the session. I say stupidly as alcohol was a big part of my smoking habit: a pint in one hand and a cigarette in the other was my normal modus operandi. I told the first friend who arrived exactly what I thought of the hypnotherapy session when he asked. 'It was a load of old rubbish,' I said. 'It didn't work. I wasn't hypnotised.'

'Pfft,' he said.

'Pfft,' I replied. 'Get the beers in.'

I said the same thing over and over again, all night long, while holding court at that bar in a pub somewhere in Soho. Each time another friend or two arrived: 'It was a load of old rubbish. It didn't work. I wasn't hypnotised. Pfft. Get the beers in.' And I got very drunk indeed.

I crawled into work the next day with a bit of a hangover, got my head down and proceeded to write about my experience. At around 11.00 a.m., one of my colleagues asked me if I wanted to step outside with her for a smoke. Instead of saying 'Yes' as usual, I said something along the lines of, 'Oh god, no thanks, I can't be bothered.' And then gasped as the whole of the night before replayed itself in my mind.

As I propped up that bar, pint in hand, every time someone asked, 'Do you want to go outside for a smoke?' I had said, 'No thanks. I can't be bothered.' Which is exactly what my hypnotherapist had suggested to me, repeatedly, in the 45 minutes of the session.

'Every time someone asks you if you want a cigarette,' he intoned, 'you will say no. You will say you can't be bothered. And then you will quickly forget that you were even asked; your mind will return to whatever it was that you were doing.' And I didn't smoke a single cigarette that night. And I was too busy telling people it hadn't worked to even notice that I wasn't smoking. I didn't even have a packet of fags or a lighter on me at work the next day as my colleague asked me to join her outside. In fact, I never smoked again.†

And, after that, I was a hypnotherapy convert.

---

* In training, I learned that this was known as a 'hypnosis halo'. More on that later.
† Well, not never exactly. Maybe once or twice, about a year later. But only to test the water as it were. Which is something you should never, ever do. Unless you really, really know what you are doing. Shh!

In fact, the hypnotherapist who stopped me smoking invited me back for a second session, during which he taught me self-hypnosis in a manner very similar to the way I will be teaching you first. It's a technique that's been handed down through the generations.

However, my own success with hypnotherapy was not what got me into studying it myself. That was down to a chance encounter with a man in a gym.

I can't do this any more!

The gym was opposite the publishing agency. Now that I wasn't smoking, I was going there almost daily.*

I had picked up a new gym buddy, a guy who had joined recently and who seemed to have a similar workout schedule to mine. We talked a little bit as we spotted each other at the various benches and on the different machines, but nothing of any depth until one day I began sounding off about work. I was fed up. Stressed. Bored of my same old, same old, nine-to-five routine and, at the grand old age of 35, suffering from a weary, work-related ennui.

'Can I make a suggestion?' said my gym buddy, who had grown bored of my moaning.

'Sure,' said I.

'Well, you've talked a hell of a lot about that hypnotherapy session you had. In fact, you still seem quite excited about it. And I haven't told you yet, but I'm a hypnotherapist too. Have you thought about that as a career?'

It turned out that he wasn't just a hypnotherapist – he was the director of development at the London College of Clinical Hypnosis (LCCH) and taught there on a regular basis.

And so, in true cutting a long story short style, I enrolled, and I trained. I learned some of but not all of the stuff that I will be sharing with you in this book. I was taught how to hypnotise people safely and I was taught, among other things, how to use hypnotherapy to help with anxiety, depression, weight control, pain control, stopping smoking and even skin conditions such as eczema and psoriasis. It also showed me how to

---

* If you get rid of a bad habit, you need to replace it with a good one, or risk an equally bad, or more bad habit creeping in. Nature abhors a vacuum after all.

help people remember where they'd left their car keys or, if they'd been particularly rambunctious, where they'd left their car.*

I later specialised in REBT (which will feature heavily in Part Three of this book). But if you want to learn a whole lot more about it, then there's a book (by me) that's all about it. Check out *The Four Thoughts That F*ck You Up (and how to fix them)* and let me know what you think.

Alongside my private practice, I worked for the NHS in the Royal Brompton Hospital, where I specialised in pain control for the best part of ten years. What I did there was quite revolutionary and certainly made its mark. I'd probably be working in the hospital still if I hadn't moved to Bristol in 2016.

Once there, I did something equally revolutionary and introduced Hypnotherapy for Stress Management on to the group therapy programme of a psychiatric hospital I began working at. I ran that successfully (alongside two other groups, one on positive psychology and the other on REBT) for more than five years.

I'm only telling you these things, laying out my credentials as it were, so that you can trust that I do know what I am on about, and that I practise clinical hypnotherapy and REBT both safely and with a great deal of experience. Believe me when I say this book can help you. Also, if you ever need help remembering where you parked your car, I am most definitely your man. But back to vaudevillian entertainment for a moment before moving on.

Being terminated with an egg whisk has not been my only brush with stage hypnosis. I once went to see the mentalist Derren Brown on stage in London on a ticket bought as a present by a friend. In this show, Derren selected his subjects by throwing spinning plastic quoits out into the audience. If one touched you, he invited you up. But you didn't have to go if you didn't want to.

As he set this up on stage, chucking quoits out left, right and centre, my friend turned to me. 'Wouldn't it be funny if one of those – oh never mind,' she whispered, as a bright red spinning disc hit me hard in the middle of my forehead. Of course, I went up.

'Hello,' said Derren, 'what's your name, and what do you do for a living?'

'Well,' I replied, 'it's funny you should ask.'

---

* I've helped three people this way: one after their wedding, one after a stag do and another after a very heavy Saturday night out in an unfamiliar town.

My career choices did not exclude me from his routine as what I do and what he does are different. He didn't even hypnotise me. Instead, I was part of a psychological trick in which he got a group of us up on stage, predicted (to the audience) which people would pick which thing and then subtly manipulated us into picking the thing he had predicted we would pick.*

In the next chapter I'm going to talk about what hypnotherapy is, how it works and exactly how it can help you. But first, I want to give you another taste of trance, and I want you to do it by staring at a wall until your eyes water.

Another taste of trance

Please sit comfortably in a chair or on your sofa. It doesn't matter where. I don't mind if you're propped up in bed or sitting on the loo, just so long as you are comfortable and are staring at a wall (or even a door opposite you).

I want you to pick a spot or a mark on the wall or door, perhaps even a crack or a shadow, and I want you to focus all your attention on it. Keep focusing. Let your vision dance, let your eyes water, let other details and aspects on the wall or door fade in and out of your awareness. When you've had enough, when your eyes feel really tired from all the eye watering and detail dancing, let them close and allow them to comfortably relax. And, as you allow your eyes to comfortably relax, let that sense of relaxation spread throughout the rest of your body. Also, with one sense closed off, I want you to become aware of the things you can pick up with your other senses. What does your inner vision pick up on? What can you feel with your body and inside your body? What can you hear, externally and internally? Allow yourself to become vitally absorbed with the things you have become aware of. You might be pleasantly surprised at how many there are. When you're ready, finish the exercise but please feel free to repeat it a few more times. Closing your eyes like this and creating this heightened state of awareness is the very beginning of trance. You'll find out why I want you to do this in the next chapter.

---

* I'd have still been a willing participant even if it had included hypnosis, so I would have gone into a trance (more on that later).

Hypnotherapy, the basics

Hypnotherapy and hypnosis are two different things, although the two words and concepts are often conflated. Hypnosis is a state of trance, while hypnotherapy is what is delivered to you in that state of trance. Hypnosis is an altered state of consciousness (that's one theory anyway) that is very similar to daydreaming or, as you discovered earlier, losing yourself in a book. The term itself is based on the Greek word *hypnos* and is a little bit of a misnomer. Hypnos is the Greek god of sleep. But with hypnosis you are somewhere between being asleep and being awake – neither one nor the other.

The term 'hypnosis' was coined by the surgeon Dr James Braid (1795–1860) and he later regretted it (more on him in Chapter 5). Hypnos was the god you called upon to get a good night's sleep. He also got the blame for anyone who fell into an unexplainable, inexplicable or just plain weird sleep-like state.[*]

Hypnotherapy, meanwhile, is therapy (or counselling or coaching) conducted in that state of hypnosis, and there are different therapies for different things depending on what it is that you want to achieve. You can have hypnotherapy for anxiety and depression, for building confidence and anger management, you can have it for weight control, pain control, stopping smoking, increasing your wellbeing, decreasing your stress, building resilience and much more.

---

[*] The Roman equivalent was Somnus, who also got blamed for odd forms of sleep, hence the term 'somnambulism', or sleepwalking.

Whatever it is you want to achieve, the seeds of it are sown during a hypnotherapy session. But we human beings drift in and out of hypnotic states of being umpteen times a day. And there are two types of trance: relaxed and focused.

Relaxing trance includes things such as daydreaming, napping (when you are dreaming and yet still aware of what is going on around you), falling asleep and waking up, and zoning out. Focused states include being in the 'zone' (athletes describe this a lot), losing yourself in a really good book, becoming so involved in work or a project that hours seem like minutes (in a state of 'flow') and, even, driving your car. If you have been driving for a good while then you will probably have had the following experience: you get in the car at point A, undertake your journey, exit the car at point B and then go, 'But I don't really remember that journey.' You then worry a little, thinking that you're a bad driver when, in fact, the opposite is true. You have become an unconsciously competent driver (more on this and how to become unconsciously competent at anything later). You are so good at driving, so focused on the art of it, that changing gears, braking, indicating, slowing down, speeding up, giving way and changing lanes blend so seamlessly, so effortlessly, that it's almost as if you aren't paying it any attention at all.

Your mind likes going into these trance-like states and it does so with a practised ease. You've been doing it since you were young; just think of all those times you were told off for not paying attention and staring meaninglessly into space. And while you're in one, a really nice thing happens to your mind (for the purposes of therapy, that is).

Before we proceed with that, there's just one thing. I hope that many of you reading this have seen *Star Wars*. Specifically *Return of the Jedi*. There's a scene where Luke Skywalker has it confirmed by Yoda that Darth Vader really is his father, meaning that his earlier mentor Ben Kenobi was a little economical with the truth about his parentage. A few minutes later, Luke meets Ben in ghostly form and chastises him. Ben says that what he told Luke was true but, 'from a certain point of view'. Luke basically responds with a 'yeah, right'. Ben goes on to explain that many truths that we cling to in life depend greatly upon our point of view. The theories of what hypnosis is and how hypnotherapy works are many and varied (as are the theories of mind). So, what I am about to tell you is true, but from a certain point of view.

Icebergs ahead!

Very simplistically, there are two parts to the mind: the conscious and the unconscious. But it's not a 50/50 split. Think of it like an iceberg in the ocean. This metaphor is mistakenly attributed to the famous psychoanalyst Sigmund Freud (1856–1939), but he never came up with it. No one really knows who did. He's the one who made the ideas about the conscious and unconscious mind famous, but he's not the one who came up with the icebergs to explain it. But it is a good analogy and Freud is stuck with it for now. With any iceberg, about 10 per cent of it is above the waterline and, therefore, visible, while the remaining 90 per cent of it is hidden below the water. Your conscious mind is the 10 per cent above the water line and is your immediate, short-term memory part of the equation. It is the part of you that remembers the phone number you only need to use once or to pick up a loaf of bread on the way home because somebody asked you to and so on, and it contains all the thoughts, feelings and memories that you are consciously aware of at any given time. It is also the rational, logical and analytical part of your mind.*

So, what do you think the unconscious part of the mind is responsible for? Go on, take a guess before reading on.

The short answer is everything else. As you read this book, you are blinking, breathing, digesting food, regulating body temperature and conducting thousands of other processes without consciously thinking about them. A lot of these things are known as autonomic body functions, and it is your unconscious mind that takes care of them for you. It is also the database of everything you are: all your thoughts and feelings and memories; everything you have ever seen and felt and done. Everything you have ever learned and witnessed and done is stored there, as are all your skills and habits (both good and bad).

Some illustrations of the mind-as-iceberg include three 'layers': the conscious, the preconscious and the unconscious. The preconscious mind consists of anything that could be brought (in theory) into the conscious mind and is really part of the unconscious mind. And, if

---

* Some people (therapists, scholars etc.) call it the unconscious and some call it the subconscious. I prefer the former over the latter.

we are going to be pedantic, the conscious mind is also technically part of the unconscious too, so really, it's just one great big iceberg both seen and unseen.

Technically, scientists believe that the unconscious is everything in the brain below the top layers of the neocortex. However, some psychologists dispute Freud's idea of the unconscious and science can't fully prove where our consciousness resides anyway (it could be the brain, it could be our cells, it could be in the ether around us) so no one really knows where the iceberg dwells.

But for now, conscious and unconscious, 10 per cent and 90 per cent. The two parts of your mind are in constant communication all day long. The conscious mind is like a reader (again, this is very simplistic, and about as accurate as the iceberg metaphor but it's enough to do the job). And it is forever checking up on how to be you. 'What do I do there?' it asks, and 'How do I feel about that?' it wonders, and 'How do I respond to them?' it questions. Check, check, check, check and check. Over and again. Except in hypnosis.

In hypnosis, that communication process is bypassed. Sort of. But not really: your conscious mind is still there, and still aware of everything going on around it but it can't quite access the unconscious mind in the same way. Left alone, the unconscious mind is very susceptible to positive suggestion, especially if those suggestions are tied to a goal you already know you want to achieve.

So, a hypnotherapist will deliver suggestions based upon your life or therapy goals while you are in a trance so that they are stored in your unconscious mind. When you come out of hypnosis and the two parts of your mind start communicating again, there's a whole barrel load of new information in there that your conscious mind will accept more readily the next time it does its check-in.

Think of it as a bit like this. Let's say you have a low opinion of yourself, and that your self-talk is quite negative. Someone will pay you a compliment, such as 'You have a nice smile,' but because your self-talk isn't that good, you will reject the compliment, won't know what to say in the face of it, and will probably just excuse it (they're just saying that to be 'nice', you'll think). You might become flustered, or angry, or both. However, with hypnotherapy, let's say the hypnotherapist has intoned, over and again, that your self-talk is good, that you like, accept and admire yourself and that you do, indeed, have a very nice smile. Well, then, the next time someone pays you a smile-related compliment, while part of you will still reject it, another part of you will accept it, think 'Yes, I do' and glow, ever so slightly, with pride. You will likely say 'Thank you' to the person who made the compliment and perhaps, even, mean it.

And that is basically it. In a nutshell. My apologies to the scientists and scholars who are choking on their cornflakes as they read this but this doesn't sound too bad now, does it?

That's how it works, but what does it feel like? Well, that, more or less, depends on you.

Everything is experiential

Very simplistically put (again, scientists, scholars and academics might want to take a little lie-down), there are three levels of trance: light, medium and deep. But what you experience isn't really an indication of what level of trance you are in anyway.

You might hear every word the hypnotherapist says and recall it with pinpoint accuracy; you might drift in and out of that conscious awareness and only remember bits and pieces. Then again, your conscious mind might decide to take a holiday and disappear for a bit, there to do its own thing (you kind of remember what the therapist is saying at the beginning and the next thing you know, they are waking you up but the bit in the middle, the therapy bit, is a complete blank to you). But it's all good. It's your conscious mind that's listening (or not), and we don't work with the conscious mind, we work with the unconscious mind. And that part of you will remember everything that is said to it, even if you don't consciously remember it.

So, the good thing here is that you don't have to actively listen to a word your hypnotherapist is saying. It can all go over your conscious head as 'blah, blah, blah' and still have an effect. You can even get lost in your various trains of thought and that is all good, too.

Hypnotherapy isn't like meditation or mindfulness. You won't be expected to clear your mind of all thoughts or focus on one thought to the exclusion of all others, or step back and observe your thoughts from a detached distance. No, bring 'em on! You'll be thinking thoughts about anything and everything. Some of them will be related to the therapy and most of them won't. If you're anything like me you'll be thinking thoughts about home life and work life, about various projects both personal and professional, social commitments and, maybe, even the shopping list for whatever supermarket you frequent. None of those thoughts will get in the way. You'll even be thinking thoughts about the experience of hypnosis.

The thing is, no two people will experience hypnosis in quite the same way, and the same person won't necessarily experience hypnosis in the same way each time.

Hypnotherapy is very comfortable and relaxing. Even when you're using focused trance for the therapy. But comfort means different things to different people and feels different for different people at different times.

Again, at its most basic, it might just feel comfortable. Comfortably sitting on the chair, comfortably leaning back on the recliner and so on (but then, when I was training, we hypnotised each other while sitting not very comfortably on plastic school chairs and it still worked). But comfort can also get deeper. Much deeper.

Some people feel like they're sinking down into the chair while others feel like they are rising up out of it. And you can feel all sorts of other things besides. So, your limbs could feel heavy, or light, or tingly, or not there at all, and that is all evidence of trance to some degree or other.

I still like taking myself off to be hypnotised by other practitioners every now and then. When I'm really relaxed in hypnosis, my arms and legs feel like they weigh a ton and can't move, my head lolls to one side. When I am really, really relaxed, I'm hardly aware of my body at all. It's like my head is floating all on its own in perfect comfort. When I get to that point, I'm in my happy place and I know that the suggestions I receive are really going to hit home. This might sound a bit weird, and it is a bit weird, but in a good way. When things get like that, the best thing to do is to just go with it.

The trick of hypnotherapy is to not analyse it too much. There will be a certain level of analysis for sure. Especially if you're trying it for the first time, but if you just accept that whatever you are thinking, whatever you are feeling, and whatever you are experiencing (head lolls and all) is totally appropriate for you as you are at that juncture and then just go with the flow, it's going to help you get the most from your hypnotherapy session.

A little bit about control

This issue of control: who has it? Will you lose it? Do you surrender it to me? These questions crop up more than any other. And not without good reason. Most people conflate stage hypnotism (hypnosis for entertainment) with hypnotherapy (hypnosis for therapeutic gain). And the former does look kind of controlling. But either way, a hypnotherapist or hypnotist has no control over you. Really, they don't. They don't even hypnotise you, for a start.

Let's say that you thought hypnosis was a load of old rubbish (both for entertainment and for therapy) and that you could not be hypnotised. You would be completely correct, and no one would be able to guide you into trance. You either allow it or you don't. People already know how to go into a trance in their day-to-day lives: nodding off, daydreaming, going into a state of flow and so on. All you do in a therapy session is allow the hypnotherapist to guide you into a trance-like state. It happens by agreement. You allow the therapist to guide you into a trance, there to conduct the therapy you have agreed upon. Even stage hypnosis happens by agreement. The stage hypnotist doesn't pick on people because that wouldn't work. No, he asks for volunteers. 'Pick me!' people cry. 'Pick me!' with their arms waving in the air, 'I want to be the entertainment, I want to be the centre of attention.'

I didn't have to go up on the stage when I was hit by Derren Brown's quoit. I went because I wanted to.

The person coming for hypnotherapy has already selected themselves for therapy via that modality. If at any point during the hypnotherapy session the therapist said something that wasn't connected with either deepening the trance to the appropriate level or helping you with the agreed-upon goals, you would be able to wake up. If they suddenly whispered, 'You want to bark like a dog' or 'You want to give me your credit card details', you would, at some point, open your eyes and say, 'You what?' It might not happen immediately, but at some point, the request, which sits at odds with your therapeutic goals, would filter thought to your conscious mind.

When a stage hypnotist gets you to bark like a dog, or reveal personal information, it is because you don't mind doing so; you have agreed upon that for the purposes of entertainment.

Either way, you are in control at all times and during all stages of the hypnotherapy session.

Let's look at a hypnotherapy session. There are five main parts:

1 The introduction

This bit is very important. The better hypnotherapy is introduced and explained, the more likely it is to be successful. It's why there's a lot of information in the introductory section of this book. In fact, it's a big reason why there is an introductory section at all. It's also the bit where the therapist finds out what your goal or goals are for the course of therapy and, even, each individual session. The better the set-up, the more relaxed about hypnosis and hypnotherapy you will be.

2 The induction

This is where you get someone to close their eyes. You usually do it by tiring their eyes out by getting them to stare at something. Sometimes, some people do it automatically, without you having to ask them; some need a little bit of coaxing to do so; and some need a whole lot of coaxing to do so. But closed eyes are comfortable eyes. They are relaxed eyes. They are eyes that belong to a mind that is now ready not only for trance, but also for the next part of the therapy session. It's why I got you to practise this in the previous chapter. If you did it a fair few times, you've already set yourself up for success.

3 The deepener

This is where the trance is deepened to the appropriate level for the therapy that is being undertaken. Some therapies require a fairly light level of trance, and some need a really deep level of trance. That said, most therapies (including most in this book) operate at the medium-to-deep level.

4 The therapy bit

This is where your life or therapy goal is weaved in and worked towards using positive suggestions, metaphors, guided imagery and more. Depending on the session (and sometimes the amount of time you have), this could take anywhere from five minutes to 45 minutes, and sometimes more. This part of the process usually includes posthypnotic suggestions (suggestions that are carried out after the session) and also ego-strengthening suggestions (generic or specific suggestions that just help you to feel better about yourself, or stronger, or calmer, or more in control).

5 The awakener

Once the therapy part is concluded, you bring the person (or you can bring yourself) out of the trance. The term itself is a little incorrect as you are not 'woken up' (you were not asleep). Instead, you are brought back from a trance to full waking consciousness.

So now you know all you really need to know to begin experiencing a proper hypnosis session. Which is timely as, in the next chapter, I will be teaching you self-hypnosis, giving you a couple of suggestions to use with it, and then asking you to commit to practising it on a regular basis. But only if you want to. Only if you agree to do so.

After all, I can't make you do anything you don't want to do, can I? But you do want to give it a go, don't you?

4

Self-hypnosis

So, we now know that hypnosis is an altered state of consciousness, very similar to daydreaming or losing yourself in a really good book. We drift in and out of these altered states of consciousness umpteen times a day.

There is nothing weird or unusual about these trance-like states at all; your mind goes there with a practised ease. It likes to go there. Self-hypnosis is simply the art of you helping yourself go into one of those altered states, at a specific time, in a specific place, and then delivering positive suggestions to yourself for purposes set by yourself.

Most people are hypno-suggestible to some degree or other. The lemon exercise from the Prologue that you tried out was one such hypno-suggestibility test. Another one involves clasping your hands together very tightly and imagining that they are glued together, stuck even. You then imagine trying to pull your stuck, glued hands apart while telling yourself that the harder you try, the more they appear stuck together. Note that even if tests such as these don't work very well for you, it doesn't mean you are not a candidate for hypnotherapy.

You remember when I said earlier that there are three levels to trance: light, medium and deep? Well, there are a few (very broad) statistics to clear up first. Here they are:

- **90 per cent** of all human beings can drift into a light trance;
- **70 per cent** of those will be able to go into a medium trance;
- **20 per cent** of those will be able to go into a deep trance.

Now, before you decide you are one of the 10 per cent who can't even get to a light trance, I just want to say who that includes. First of all, it includes all those people who think hypnosis is a load of old rubbish and that they cannot be hypnotised (and they're right, remember). But this also includes people with drug and alcohol problems at the serious end of the scale, as they are already in an altered state of consciousness. We're talking a bottle of whiskey a day people or a couple of grams of something white and powdery a night people.

Some books make self-hypnosis seem ever so complicated, but it's not. It can be quite involved but it can also be quite brief.

The hypnotherapist who stopped me smoking taught me self-hypnosis and he did it briefly. I was later taught self-hypnosis again on the course I studied at the London College of Clinical Hypnosis. This version, too, was equally brief. And so, with the above firmly in mind, the technique I teach you here will be just as brief. But there is a big ask upfront, and it's a bit of a chore.

In order for self-hypnosis to be a lifelong tool, there for you to access whenever you need it, it needs to be firmly embedded in your mind as a 'thing'. You will find out in Chapter 6 why 'practice makes perfect' can be backed up by science. For it to be firmly embedded in your mind as a thing, you will need to practise self-hypnosis regularly and often.

In the beginning, it needs to be practised twice a day, every day for a good ten days or so and, after that, preferably daily (or at least a few times a week) for another 11 days. Once you have done this for a good three weeks, it is reasonably safe to assume that self-hypnosis has become embedded in your unconscious mind, and that you have the beginnings of your hypnotherapy habit. After that, you are free to use it as and when you see fit on the tacit understanding that, within two to eight months it will be an ingrained, habitual behaviour and that, eventually, with further practice still, you will be a self-hypnosis guru.

Repetition is not only important for mastering the art of self-hypnosis, it's also an essential element of every topic and exercise in this book – because it's not self-hypnosis per se that counts (although it can, and you'll find out how in the case study on the next page) but what you do with it.

Before we go any further, I just want to remind you that hypnosis is completely safe, with no harmful side effects whatsoever. You are in control of your mind at all times, and you won't get 'stuck' in a hypnotic state. The worst thing that can happen is that you might nod off, so perhaps consider where you are practising. This might especially happen if you do it in bed last thing at night. If you do that, please make sure that you also practise at some other point during the day (sitting in a comfortable chair). If you only practise in bed at night, it can become a great tool for a good night's sleep (ten, nine, eight, zzzz) but not much else.

How to practise self-hypnosis

The following bullet-point instructions are a cross between what the stop smoking hypnotherapist taught me and what I learned on my hypnotherapy course. It's how I practise self-hypnosis to this day.

- Sit in a comfortable chair, somewhere quiet, where you have a reasonable chance of being undisturbed.
- Stare at a spot on the wall opposite (as you did earlier) until your eyes feel like they want to close.
- Close your eyes.
- Take a few deep breaths and allow yourself to relax.
- Take a moment to acknowledge the normal, everyday sounds around you (none of them will disturb you; in fact, they will just become part of the overall experience).
- Silently, mentally, count down from ten on each out breath until you reach the number one.
- Between each two or three numbers, tell yourself 'I am becoming more deeply and deeply relaxed' (ten, nine – deeper and deeper relaxed – eight, seven, six – deeper and deeper relaxed – five, four, three – deeper and deeper relaxed – two, one – and all the way, deep down, relaxed).
- When you reach the number one, safely assume that you are in a trance to some degree or other.
- Give yourself positive, beneficial suggestions.
- Stay in hypnotic trance for as long as you wish.
- When you are ready, slowly count up from one to ten.
- Open your eyes.
- That's it.

A little bit more detail

It really does pay to sit in a very comfortable chair. At least, in the beginning. You can sit in an uncomfortable chair if you wish, and it will still work (I practised in that classroom while sitting on those plastic chairs for over a year-and-a-half), but a comfy chair helps you to relax almost immediately. It's best not to lie down, as you're more likely to nod off. Turn the heating up if you wish, drape a blanket over yourself if you don't. Do anything that helps you to feel warm and snuggly. When you are comfortable, just pick a spot, or a mark, or a crack, or a crease in the wallpaper on the wall opposite you and stare at it intently. Keep staring until your eyes begin to tire and, when they do, simply close your eyes. With your eyes comfortably closed, you will need to count down from ten to one silently, mentally. Do this in a slow, sleepy, monotone voice in your brain. The sort of voice you would use to send a child to sleep. Also, and this is a very important bit, time the countdown with your out breath. When you breathe in, you naturally tense up but when you breathe out, you naturally let every little bit of you relax more. So, when you time your countdown with each out breath, you are helping to facilitate that descent into relaxation. You might even want to count down on each second out breath to really slow things down.

When you reach the number one, just trust that you are in a trance to some degree or other. As mentioned in the previous section, there are three levels of trance (light, medium and deep) and what you experience is not necessarily an indication of what level you're at, so just trust that you are in a hypnotic trance, even if it doesn't feel anything like what you want or are expecting. Also, at this point, the most important thing is that you practise, practise, practise; even if you don't think you are in a trance.

When you have reached the number one, you can either allow yourself to drift in that state of trance for as long as you wish (five minutes, ten or 15, even 20 minutes if you like), or you can give yourself positive, beneficial suggestions.

A positive suggestion is where you say something that you do want as opposed to something you don't want. For instance, if I said to you right now, 'Don't think about the big, pink elephant,' then all you will be able to see in your mind's eye is a big, pink, dancing elephant.*

This is because, for the mind to negate something, it must first accept it. So, 'Don't think about the big, pink elephant' accepts the big, pink elephant. In a similar fashion, saying 'I must not fail' accepts the possibility of failure, so failure is what your mind will focus on, while

* It is dancing now that I've said it is dancing.

saying 'I will not be anxious' is accepting and therefore allowing for your anxiety. Instead, try saying things such as 'I will succeed' and 'I am calm and in control'. At this point, don't overload yourself, just pick three positive suggestions that you would like to repeat to yourself over and over again, like a mantra. Common suggestions include:

- 'Every day, I am becoming more confident.'
- 'Every day, I feel calmer and more in control.'
- 'Every morning, I wake feeling refreshed and energised.'

Repeat these suggestions (in your head, not out loud) for as long as you like, but when you are ready, or whenever the thought pops in your mind, simply count up from one to ten and, when you reach the number ten, open your eyes. Whenever you open your eyes, you will be fully returned to whatever room you are in, and all normal sensations will return to your eyes and limbs. Pretty soon, you'll be replacing those mantras with the scripts in this book.

People often ask if they will fall asleep when they practise self-hypnosis or stay in a trance for longer than they wished. I'll address the latter concern first. Do you wake up a second or two before your alarm clock goes off in the morning? Chances are, you probably do. Our unconscious minds are very good at knowing what the time is, at any given time of the year, so if you regularly wake up to an alarm at 7.00 a.m., you'll often find that your mind wakes you up just before the alarm goes off. And, although I've asked you to practise self-hypnosis in a comfy chair, somewhere you won't be disturbed, I've taught people to practise self-hypnosis while they are on the toilet at work or on the Tube, train or bus on the way to work. And, as far as I know, no one has ever missed a meeting or gone past their stop. Before you start your self-hypnosis session, just instruct your unconscious mind. Tell it, 'I will stay in a trance for 15 minutes only' or, 'I will come out of the trance just before such-and-such station'. You will be pleasantly surprised to find that you will start to come out of the trance almost exactly at the 15-minute mark or right before your train enters the station. And as for the former, as mentioned earlier, if you practise in bed, you probably will nod off (just make sure you're not only using it as a sleep aid). Very rarely will you nod off when you practise during the day but, if you do, it won't be sleep, it won't be deep, and you will rouse yourself, quickly. At that point, you can either carry on repeating your positive suggestions, or you can end the session there and then and get on with your day.

1. 'Self-hypnosis' script (if you want to record yourself)

These days, practically every one of us has either a smartphone or a tablet, or a smartphone and a tablet. Said devices almost always contain a voice memo or voice recording app, so it's very easy for you to record yourself speaking the scripts in this book on to your device and then play them back. Remember to keep your voice calm and steady as you do so; slow, but not too slow, as well as a little flat and monotone (although you can slightly emphasise key words and suggestions). The dots between the words in the script below (and all other scripts in this book) indicate a comfortable pause, just a few seconds long.

Make yourself comfortable ... sit in that chair ... arms resting comfortably by your side ... or on your lap ... or on the arms of the chair ... feet flat on the ground ... and begin to stare at a mark ... or a spot ... or a shadow ... on the wall opposite ... keep staring, allow your eyes to feel heavy and tired ... heavy and tired ... so heavy and tired that they are wanting to close ... so just let them close ... close those eyes ... and allow them to remain comfortably closed ... so comfortably closed that they won't bother to open at all ... until the end of this recording ... and as you begin to relax ... it's perfectly fine for you to be aware of all the sounds around you ... all the normal, everyday sounds around you will not disturb you, they will simply fade into the background, and in some strange way, simply help you to relax more and more deeply as you go on ... and so in a few moments ... you will hear yourself count down from ten to one ... and with each descending number between ten and one ... you are going to go ten times more deeply relaxed ... 10 per cent more deeply relaxed ... with each descending number ... and if ... while you are counting ... you experience a slight ... though very pleasant sensation ... as if you were floating, floating down ... it only means you are drifting into that ever-deepening state of physical as well as mental relaxation ... so ready ... ten ... nine ... deeper and deeper ... eight ... seven ... six ...

deeper and deeper relaxed ... five ... four ... three ... deeper and deeper and deeper still ... two ... one ... and all the way, deep down relaxed ... and now that you are deeply relaxed, you are going to teach yourself self-hypnosis ... you are going to give yourself instructions for self-hypnosis ... and those instructions are going to embed themselves deeply into your unconscious mind, fix themselves there permanently ... and exert a great influence over you each time you practise ... and all you need to do to enter this wonderfully relaxed state is sit in a comfortable chair ... somewhere quiet ... where you have a reasonable chance of being undisturbed ... you fix your eyes on a spot or a mark on the wall opposite ... and you stare at it intently ... until your eyes tire and want to close ... so let them close ... and allow them to remain comfortably closed ... so comfortably closed that they won't bother to open at all until you wake yourself ... and with your eyes comfortably closed, you silently, mentally, count down from ten to one, just like you heard earlier ... and just like before ... each descending number between ten and one ... will help you to go ten times more deeply relaxed ... you count slowly ... on each out breath ... or maybe every second out breath ... to really slow you down ... and when you reach the number one, you will be as deeply relaxed as you are now ... you may even go much deeper ... because each time you practise ... you become more proficient ... you become more accomplished ... and when you reach the number one ... you give yourself positive, beneficial suggestions only, because the unconscious part of your mind does not like, and will not accept ... negative ... harmful ... suggestions ... you can stay in hypnosis for as long as you wish ... five minutes ... ten ... 20 ... as long as you wish ... but, whenever you are ready ... whenever a thought instructs you to do so ... you silently ... mentally ... count yourself up from one to ten ... and, as you do so ... you become more and more awake with each ascending number ... and when you reach the number one ... you will open your eyes ... and whenever you open your eyes ... you will awake refreshed and alert ... all normal sensations will return to your eyes and limbs ... and you will be fully returned to whatever room you are in ... so ready? One ... two ... three ... waking up ... waking up ... four ... five ... six ... waking up now ... seven ... eight ... open those eyes now ... nine ... and ten ... fully ... fully, wide awake ...

TOP TIPS FOR SELF-HYPNOSIS

Schedule specific times for your self-hypnosis (especially during the first three weeks) and try your best to stick to those times.
Keep up your practice (it's how you become competent and then masterful).

TOP TIPS FOR POSITIVE SUGGESTIONS

Start small: pick two or three simple suggestions.
Repeat them several times, over and over again, like a mantra, for maximum effect.
Say them softly (again in your head), but with conviction.
Use images as you give yourself suggestions (so if you are using suggestions to improve confidence, see yourself as that confident person; if you are using suggestions to become calmer and in control, again, imagine what that would look like and feel like for you).

Listen to the sound of my voice

For those of you who prefer your hypnotherapy old-school (i.e. delivered into your head, through your ears, via a hypnotherapist), then flick back to page 8 for your QR code. Scan it to listen to a hypnotherapy recording of me teaching you self-hypnosis. I've even included some suggestions to boost your confidence and improve your mood, because I'm nice like that.

Look out for this symbol throughout the book and return to page 8 to scan the QR code.

Malcolm's miracle

Practising self-hypnosis regularly is how you're going to get good at it. Practising it regularly is how you're going to master the art of adding positive suggestions to your self-hypnosis sessions so that you can achieve all that you want to achieve. However, self-hypnosis without positive suggestions can be a powerful force for healing in and of itself. I always remember one gentleman, Malcolm, who came to see me in my early days of practising at the Royal Brompton Hospital. He had been living with a condition known as cardiac syndrome X (CSX) for more than 15 years. CSX is chest pain in the absence of any coronary abnormalities. The heart and its blood vessels are fine and yet, there is pain. He arrived at my clinic stooped and exhausted, his face etched with pain. Although the pain was debilitating, he had done his best to not let it stop him. On top of that, he was one of life's doers and a people pleaser to boot. Always doing things for others – odd jobs, DIY, dishing out advice – not only for his immediate family, but also his extended family, his friends and work colleagues. Basically, he never stopped. His wife was like it too, apparently; they very rarely had any time to call their own. The first time the chest pain hit he thought he was having a heart attack. Paramedics were called. As he was strapped into the gurney and lifted into the ambulance, he was still issuing commands and dishing out advice to the people around him. One of the paramedics had to tell him to shut up.

We didn't do much in our first session. He told me his history of a life lived with the syndrome and I taught him self-hypnosis. 'How often should I practise this?' he asked. Twice a day, I told him. 'How long for?' was his next question. I told him that five minutes would be good, that ten would be better, 15 even better still, 20 would be great and that 30 minutes would be absolutely amazing. And off he went. The next week, an almost different man breezed into my clinic and wafted into my chair. His face looked fresh and his eyes alert. The stoop had gone. 'I don't know what you've done to me,' he said, 'but I feel so much better.' I didn't know what I'd done to him either as, therapeutically speaking, I hadn't done anything. Upon investigation, it turned out that Malcolm had followed my instructions to the letter. He had practised self-hypnosis twice a day, every day, and had plumped for the maximum 30 minutes.

More importantly, his friends, family and colleagues, knowing how important these sessions were going to be for his condition, actually left him alone and prevented others from interrupting him. For the first time in decades, Malcolm had two 30-minute sessions of pure relaxation all to himself, without the needs and demands of others intruding upon his time. Those two 30-minute sessions of self-hypnosis were enough to significantly kick-start his process of healing.

Who knows what you will achieve with practice? I'd be surprised if it was as life-enhancing as it was for Malcolm in your first week of trying it, but I would not be at all surprised if you were to notice several improvements.

Perhaps you'd like to watch out for them and even note them down as I talk you through the colourful history of hypnotherapy and yes, the bloke with the mad, staring eyes is in it.

A very brief history of hypnotherapy

Hypnotherapy is one of the oldest forms of healing known to man. It definitely goes back hundreds of years and sort of goes back thousands of years. Think of this as the whistle-stop tour, touching down on the prominent parts only. My apologies to all the names I've missed along the way (for they are many but space is sparce).

Once upon a time

A long time ago and in lands both near and far, far away, ecstatic trance, ecstatic dance and other altered states of consciousness for both psychological and physiological healing belonged to cultures all over the world (and, in some cases, still do). They can be found in shamanic practices and other psycho-spiritual healing modalities that go back almost as far as humanity itself (approximately 200,000 years or so). Lulling people into a trance and invoking therapeutic transformation, however, can be traced back to Ancient Egypt and, from there, to Ancient Greece.

So, come back with me some 4000 years to the time of Imhotep (yes, he of *The Mummy* fame but, fear ye not, as his name means 'he who comes in peace'). Imhotep was a priest. And a famous one at that. He was a vizier, a physician and an advisor to the pharaoh of the time (Zoah). He built the first ever pyramid in Egypt, the Step Pyramid. Not himself, obviously. He had slaves for that. But he kick-started the whole shebang. He was also a keen advocate of the sleep temple. Later Egyptians worshipped him and dedicated said sleep temples to him. A sleep temple was a healing sanctuary (heavy on the sandstone, heavy on the incense and heavy on the chanting) used to help people overcome all sorts of physical and mental problems.*

In fact, there are hieroglyphs found in several ancient Egyptian tombs and excavations that are understood to show worshippers experiencing hypnotic states (hovering ibis, reclining pharaoh, wiggly serpent singing 'Trust in Me').†

The sufferer was guided into trance with invocations, rituals and beneficial suggestions. The temple priests and priestesses would then try to ascertain and interpret their patient's apparently god-given dreams and mutterings, and through them, effect or attempt to find a cure for their ailments.

This practice later spread to Greece. There, a healer called Asclepius took over the role of Imhotep and became so mythic in quality that he was later revered as a god. In his temples, a person was placed in a sacred space or animal skin (called a *klinè*), there to be healed in a trance. Asclepius had many children. Two of his daughters were called Hygieia and Panacea. So, now you know where we get our words clinic, hygiene and, erm, panacea from.

Asclepius was possessed of a staff, a snake-entwined stick that forms part of the logo for the World Health Organization today. A double-snaked variant, carried by Hermes, the herald of the Greek gods, is a well-known medical symbol the world over.

However, while these forms of healing involved hypnosis, they weren't hypnotherapy as we understand it today. That came much, much later.

Ooh, he was so mesmeric

The understanding of modern hypnosis started with Franz Anton Mesmer (1734–1815). He was a German physician with an interest in astronomy and was, by all accounts, a bit of a character. He believed

---

* A vizier is a term for a high-ranking official in many Middle Eastern countries.
† I'm joking with my translation of the hieroglyphs, obviously. That song is pretty hypnotic though.

that both astronomy and magnets could influence our health. During an experiment with magnets in 1774 on a woman with hysteria, he perceived a fluid flowing through her body – one that could be influenced by both the magnets and his willpower. He dubbed the fluid and its manipulation 'animal magnetism' but later ditched the magnets in favour of fluid manipulation by his will alone. His theories laid the foundations for what we understand of hypnosis and trance today. His sessions (and his performances) were often very theatrical; he would stare at his subjects intently, and cloaks, mirrors, lights and music were used to good effect, as was his tone of voice.

He gave rise to the 'mesmerism' movement, and its practitioners were known as 'mesmerists'. At one point, Mesmer was so sought-after that he couldn't treat people individually and so saw them en masse in a chamber of his own devising. Known as a 'baquet', it could seat about 20 people at any one time. So, Mesmer is quite possibly the founding father of group hypnotherapy.

His practices and his movement were later discredited by an investigation initiated by King Louis XVI, but some people still believe in animal magnetism, even today. They can usually be found swathed in cheap aftershave, staring at you intently across crowded rooms. And it's because of Mesmer that the word 'mesmerising' means to transfix, or completely capture someone's attention. However, even today, 'mesmerising' (and all the theatricality that word entails) is still sometimes used as a term to describe hypnosis. While Mesmer is responsible for the myth that hypnosis is all about mad staring eyes, the next guy is responsible for the thing about the swinging pocket watches.

This won't hurt at all

Dr James Braid was a surgeon and an expert in the treatment of clubbed feet, knocked knees, curved spines, squinty eyes and more. And it was he who first coined the term 'hypnosis' but later regretted it as what he was proposing had nothing to do with sleep or with the Greek god of it, but by the time he realised his error, the name had stuck. The misnomer itself is an abbreviation of 'neuro-hypnosis' ('nervous sleep').*

* In English, at least. The French mesmerist Baron Étienne Félix d'Henin de Cuvillers used the terms *hypnotique*, *hypnotisme* and *hypnotiste* as early as 1820 but he meant them in a magnetic sense, as opposed to Braid's psychological sense.

He became interested in the subject in 1841 after attending a show by animal magnetism enthusiast Charles Lafontaine (1803–1892).

Braid's ideas of hypnosis – that it wasn't caused by magnets or willpower but instead was achieved through the vision and concentration of the subject – was a direct rejection of mesmerism. 'I adopted the term hypnotism to prevent my being confounded with those who entertain those extreme notions that a mesmeriser's will has an irresistible power over his subjects,' he said.

He found that staring at things created a hypnotic state, which is why many old-time hypnotists used a swinging pendulum (ergo, a pocket watch on a chain).

Braid was also a self-proclaimed pioneer of hypno-surgery (surgery where the patient is sedated with hypnotherapy rather than traditional anaesthetics and yes, this is a thing, even today). He was also an advocate of chemical anaesthetics (which were in their infancy). The first reliable example of a general anaesthetic being used for surgery was by a doctor in Japan in 1804. Before this it was either nothing at all or a bottle of something 70 per cent proof and a very big stick to bite on.

He is regarded by many as the first genuine hypnotherapist and/or the father of modern hypnotherapy.

Did someone say Freud?

Just as you can't mention psychotherapy without referencing Sigmund Freud, the same is true for the history of hypnotherapy. Yes, the father of psychoanalysis and the grandaddy of mummy issues (and the originator of the Oedipus Complex) was also a keen hypnotherapist, for a while at least.

He first came across it in a clinical setting when studying in Paris in 1885 under Professor Jean-Martin Charcot (1825–1893), who was using it as part of his work on hysteria. Freud later collaborated with physician Josef Breuer (1842–1925), who also used hypnosis on hysteria. Clearly, there was a lot of it about in the 1800s. However, Freud soon rejected hypnosis in favour of his own approach: conscious psychoanalysis.

Some say he rejected it because he found his suggestions didn't 'stick', while others claimed it was because he couldn't build the rapport necessary for hypnotherapy to work properly or, even more cuttingly, that it was because he was just a rubbish hypnotherapist. Ouch!

What are you even doing?

Dr Milton Erickson (1901–1980) was a prominent American psychiatrist and psychotherapist. He encouraged self-exploration in his therapy practice and took the then unconventional point of view that the patient's past wasn't necessarily the focal point for change.

Erickson was a great example of 'looking on the bright side'. He had dyslexia, was colour blind and tone-deaf. He said that these 'disabilities' allowed him to focus on aspects of communication and behaviour overlooked by most people. In therapy, this is known as emphasising the positive.

He became interested in hypnosis at an early age after seeing a sideshow hypnotist but always thought hypnosis could have better applications. At 17, he contracted polio and, stuck in bed, barely able to talk and even less able to move, began exploring the self-healing potential of it on himself. Not only did he use it to heal his ailing body (he was eventually able to talk and walk, albeit with the use of a cane), but this convalescence also allowed him to become a keen-eyed student of human behaviour and body language.

In some circles, he is considered yet another father of modern hypnotherapy. (Sadly, as we tiptoe through its history, it becomes apparent that there are far too many fathers and not nearly enough mothers of the subject.)

Hypnotherapists, up until this point, had mainly made use of direct suggestions, delivered in an authoritarian style, while Erickson made use of a more permissive, indirect and agreeable style.

This is an example of a direct suggestion: 'You will stop eating chocolate. You will stop eating chocolate right now and you are going to feel really good about the fact that you stop eating chocolate right now.'

And this is an example of an indirect suggestion: 'I wonder when you will stop eating chocolate. Maybe it will be as soon as this session has finished, or maybe tomorrow morning or, even, the afternoon. I don't know when that will be exactly, but whenever you decide to stop eating chocolate, you might even notice that you feel really good about doing so.'

Some people have become a little confused by his approach over time and say he was only ever indirect and permissive when, in fact, he could also be quite direct and authoritarian in his way. However, some professionals wonder if he even practised hypnotherapy at all since his overall approach to it was quite sublime and conversational at times.

Honourable mentions

The following really do deserve more space, but needs must and all that: James Esdaile (1808–1859), a surgeon, mesmerist and notable figure in the history of anaesthesia; the aforementioned Jean-Martin Charcot, a French neurologist, pioneer of hypnosis for hysteria, taught Freud; Hippolyte Bernheim (1840–1919), also French, a physician and neurologist who developed the theory of suggestibility in hypnotism; Émile Coué (1857–1926), a psychologist and pharmacist, introduced a popular method of psychotherapy and self-improvement based on optimistic autosuggestion (Coué is the man responsible for the infamous affirmation, 'every day, in every way, I'm getting better and better'); Edith Klemperer (1898–1987), another pioneer, but this time for the psychotherapeutic use of hypnosis; Ernest Hilgard (1904–2001), famous for research on hypnosis on pain control; Josephine Hilgard (1906–1989), developmental psychologist, hypnotherapist, wife of Ernest Hilgard (their book, *Hypnosis in the Relief of Pain*, is a must-read for anyone working in this area); Ernest Rossi (1933–2020), pioneer of mind-body healing, worked with Milton Erickson for eight years.

And that's it for the very brief history of hypnotherapy. I hope you enjoyed it and have been practising your self-hypnosis while doing so. Please carry on as, in the next chapter, before moving on to hypnotherapy proper, I want to talk you through a few things that will help you to develop not only the practice of self-hypnosis and hypnotherapy, but also the practice of anything you set your mind to. Now, how does that sound?

Little life hacks

When it comes to therapy (or life, or business, or anything for that matter), I find it helps to know a few things about the human mind, especially in relation to how we get good at anything, how our brain adapts to new information, how to build a successful habit and stick with it, and how to develop and work towards a goal. So, in this chapter, that's exactly what I'm going to talk about. Believe me, if you don't know it already, this stuff will stand you in good stead throughout both the rest of this book and the rest of your life.

The four stages of competency

Also known as the conscious competence learning mode (or how to get good at anything), this relates to the psychological stages involved in the process of progressing from incompetence to mastery in any kind of skill or ability. Those four stages are:

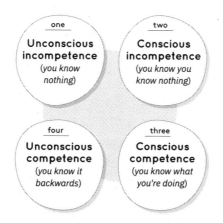

THE FOUR STAGES OF COMPETENCY

We all have different skills, and we will be at a different stages of competence with any of those skills at any given time. And most (but not all) of our skills require practice if we are to remain competent. A management trainer called Martin M. Broadwell first described this model in 1969. It was then elaborated on in 1973 in a book called *The Dynamics of Life Skills Coaching* by Paul R. Curtiss and Phillip W. Warren. It was also popular as a training model throughout the 1970s. So, let's take a closer look at that diagram.

1 Stage one: unconscious incompetence

You are rubbish at something. You might not know, or understand, or even recognise that you are. At this point, you might not even value the skill you're no good at. The amount of time spent in this stage depends on how much you want the skill.

2 Stage two: conscious incompetence

You recognise the value of the skill and your deficiency in this area. You might not know what to do or how to do it, but you want to do it, and so you commit to learning the skill, accepting the frustrations and mistakes that you will make along the way.

3 Stage three: conscious competence

Alright, so you've been putting the practice in. You know what to do now, but you do have to think about it, and you still need to put the practice in, but you're getting there.

4 Stage four: unconscious competence

You have put so much practice in that this skill has become second nature to you. You're a whizz, a pro; you can do your thing without even thinking about it. In fact, you can probably do it with your eyes closed, or while you are doing something else.

I like to compare this to driving. Before my first ever driving lesson, I was rubbish at driving, but didn't know that I was. This was my unconscious incompetence. I'd been go-kart racing several times and thought that a car would be just like that. How wrong I was. In my first driving lesson, I was all over the place. I veered too far to the left then too far to the right; I went too slow; I went too fast, and I stalled the car several times. But I vowed to continue because, as a 17-year-old, I wanted the freedom and maturity a set of wheels represented. For the next several weeks and lessons I was consciously incompetent. I knew I was rubbish but that with each lesson I would get a little better. I made mistakes and I learned from them.

I passed my test, got a car and was allowed on the road. I wasn't the best driver in the world, but I wasn't the worst either. I had to think about what I was doing, and I had to pay close attention, but I knew what I was doing. I was consciously competent but, at some point, I couldn't tell you when exactly, I became unconsciously competent. I stopped thinking about it and just did it automatically. From that point on, I changed gears, checked mirrors, indicated where necessary, slowed down and sped up accordingly, and executed all those other driving skills unconsciously and effortlessly. When you are unconsciously competent you do still need to be aware, however, as bad habits can creep in (not always keeping both hands on the steering wheel is one of mine). But the lesson here is, if you want to get good at anything, you just need to keep doing it. Your brain will help you, which is where the concept of neuroplasticity comes in.

The brain and neuroplasticity

You know that expression, 'You can't teach an old dog new tricks'? Well, it's total rubbish. Because you can teach dogs of any age, from puppy to senior, any trick you want and it cares to learn.

Not only is it rubbish, but the saying itself is based on an expression made popular (in 1546 no less!) by the writer John Heywood. However, he was referencing an even earlier treatise: the *Boke of Husbandry* (a then agricultural classic written in 1523 by the English judge, scholar and legal author, Sir Anthony Fitzherbert). In it, he wrote that, 'the dogge must lerne it, whan he is a whelpe, or els it will not be: for it is harde to make an olde dogge to stoupe.'

For those of you who don't speak Olde English, Fitzherbert was saying that a dog needs to learn when it is a new puppy or else it will be hard for him to comply. And we've been stuck with this idiom ever since, despite the amount of evidence to the contrary (this is a well-researched area, not only on dogs but also on people).

When it comes to us, scientists once thought that the brain's structure was hard-wired and immutable. The consensus was that the brain was a machine: capable of many things, programmable when young, but not capable of change or growth. But then modern research showed up – with its fancy magnetic resonance imaging (MRI), computerised tomography (CT) and positron emission tomography (PET) scans – and showed us that the brain is actually plastic. Not literally. You're not going to die and pollute the Earth with your brain for the next 450 years.*

The term refers to neural plasticity. The brain is malleable; it can change, grow and develop based upon the experiences and stimuli you give it. Even in old age! The adult brain retains this neuroplasticity and can change both shape and function.

The brain is made up of neurons, millions of nerve cells that make up our so-called 'grey matter'. These neurons process and transmit information through electrical and chemical signals. There are about 86 billion of them in the human brain.

The production of these neurons is known as neurogenesis and while it slows down as we get older, making our brains less malleable, it is a process that carries on throughout our entire lifespan. This means that a brain can not only adapt to the challenges inflicted on it via damage, but also learn to cope with any changes and experiences it encounters as it goes through life.

The more often you do something, the more often a neural pathway will fire, and the stronger the connections become. This is called long-term potentiation and is important (to my mind at least) to not only what we've just discussed regarding competency, but also to the building of habits (see below). And it is very important for hypnotherapy. Neurogenesis will occur when you are learning a new instrument. It will also occur when you imagine learning a new instrument in, say, a hypnotic trance.

And that's not all. Let's say you work out down the gym. You know that expression, 'practice makes perfect?' Well, that one is not a load of old rubbish. Not only will practice help you become unconsciously competent, but it will also build stronger neural pathways based upon everything you do down the gym. You also build stronger muscles, obviously. Studies have also demonstrated that if you imagine a gym workout in hypnotherapy, not only will you build stronger neural pathways, but also stronger muscles. They will get stronger. Not as strong

---

* Which is roughly how long it takes for plastic to decompose in landfill.

as if it were an actual workout, but there would still be a significant increase in muscle mass.

In fact, hypnosis has a strong track record in improving many aspects of exercise and sports performance.

Doing things changes the structure of your brain. Never picked up a violin before? Never studied music? Well, it doesn't matter if you are seven, 17 or 72 – the minute you pick up an instrument, the minute you start learning to play it, the minute you start to read music, new neurons will fire, your brain will change shape, form and function based upon this new information and those neural networks will only get stronger with practice. For instance:

- A London black cab driver typically has a larger hippocampus than the average human brain and stores a more detailed map of the city. The study of this map is called The Knowledge.
- Musicians have 130 per cent more grey matter in the auditory cortex than the average human brain.
- Meditating monks, especially those meditating on compassion, have an abundance of activity in the left prefrontal cortex, as opposed to the right, giving an increased capacity for joy and a reduced propensity for negativity.

Obviously, there is a downside to neurogenesis. Those who ruminate negatively and worry excessively will build wicked worry brains, awesome anxiety brains or dexterous depression brains. But the good news is that you can fire new neurons, build new networks and, with regular practice, build happier, healthier brains.

Research has shown that you can improve neuroplasticity by enriching your environment (learning a new language, picking up an instrument, visiting new places, reading etc.), getting good sleep on a nightly basis, exercising regularly, meditating often and playing games.

How long does it take to build a habit?

The American essayist, philosopher and historian Will Durant (1885–1981) once famously wrote, 'We are what we repeatedly do. Excellence, then, is not an act, but a habit.' Once we repeatedly do something, our unconscious mind will take care of it for us. What was once a conscious act becomes an unconscious one; it becomes habitual. As complicated as we like to think we are, we are basically just a collection of habits. But just how long does it take to build a habit?

When asked, most people say it takes 21 days. This idea most likely originated with prominent plastic surgeon, Dr Maxwell Maltz (1899–1975), and his book, *Psycho-Cybernetics*. Published in 1960, it's based on the theory that you can programme your mind to achieve things, such as success and happiness, in the same way you'd programme a machine. When talking about his various exercises, Maltz wrote, 'these, and many other commonly observed phenomena, tend to show that it requires a minimum of about 21 days for an old mental image to dissolve and a new one to gel.'

The book sold more than 30 million copies but, sadly, in its popularity, most people leapt on the '21' part of that quote and not on the 'minimum' part, and thus a myth was born. In fact, when I was taught hypnotherapy for stopping smoking, I was told that if someone starts smoking within the first three weeks after the session, the treatment hasn't worked. So, you see them for free, find out what went wrong and fix it. However, if they smoke after three weeks or more have elapsed, then they made a conscious decision to break their new non-smoking habit. You can invite them back and work with that decision but you charge them again.

However, according to a 2009 study published in the *European Journal of Social Psychology*, it takes anywhere from 18 to 254 days for a person to form a new habit. From their research, the authors also concluded that it takes an average of 66 days for a new behaviour to become automatic.

You can certainly build a new habit in just 21 days, but it will be just that, 'new'. It will be like a tiny little shoot appearing out of the ground. For that shoot to become stronger, more robust and more connected to all the other shoots around it – for it to be considered truly automatic and habitual – it's safer to aim for the 66-day end of the spectrum and beyond.

But whether you take the view that it's 21 days, 66 days or 254 days, the best way to build a habit is to stick to it and the best way to stick to it is to have a very clear goal in mind, which brings me to the last topic in this section.

'Cos you want goals

Psychotherapy (and coaching, and business for that matter) make good use of what is known as SMART goals. A SMART goal is one that is Specific, Measurable, Achievable, Relevant and Time-bound.

So, for instance, saying you want to get fitter isn't SMART. It's a goal, definitely, but it's not specific enough. How fit do you want to be? How are you going to measure this? What is your timeframe?

Specific can also mean simple, sensible, meaningful and significant, while Measurable can also mean meaningful and motivating. Achievable, meanwhile, can also mean agreed on and attainable; Relevant can mean reasonable, realistic and resourced and/or results based; and Time-bound can mean time-based, time-limited, timely and time-sensitive.

So, saying you want to 'get fitter' does not fulfil the above criteria and is therefore not SMART. Nor does saying you want to get fitter in two weeks. Now, saying you want to get fitter over the next 14 weeks so that you can complete a parkrun 5k race (or another sporting challenge that appeals to you) is a SMART goal as it ticks every box and allows for an achievable and healthy improvement in fitness.

So, as you approach the advice and hypnotherapy scripts in this book, please do develop SMART goals for whatever it is you want to achieve. However, there's another way for you to achieve your goals – one that is a little easier and for which all you need to do is make a wish. It's called a WOOP goal. An evidence-based strategy developed by Gabriele Oettingen and her husband, Peter Gollwitzer, at New York University, it's proven to be highly effective. WOOP stands for:

W   Wish
O   Outcome
O   Obstacle
P   Plan

So, you make a wish (set a goal, state an intention) and announce the outcome (why it's a good goal for you). You then think about the potential obstacle or obstacles and develop a plan or solution, should that obstacle occur.

This is a WOOP goal a client of mine set herself:

Wish: To be more focused on the days when I work from home.

Outcome: I will be more productive and feel happier about that.

Obstacle: I have too many distractions (mobile phone, tablet, television) that mean I procrastinate and delay the start of my working day.

Plan: When I know I am working from home the next day, the night before I will turn my mobile phone and tablet off and lock them in a kitchen drawer along with the TV remote. The first and only electronic device I will turn on in the morning will be my work laptop.

Research has shown that setting a WOOP goal is way more successful than, say, just stating an intention, or expressing an affirmation. Its success lies in the use of mental contrasting (as in it gets you to contrast a wish with an inner obstacle and then create an if/then solution).

Now you have everything you need to make really good use of the rest of this book. Part Two is all about using hypnotherapy to enhance various aspects of your wellbeing. The technique I'm going to talk you through first is not only another great way to practise self-hypnosis, but it is also an essential stressbusting tool. It's also part of a method for falling asleep fast. Not bad, eh?

PART
TWO

ENHANCE YOUR WELLBEING WITH HYPNOTHERAPY

7

What is wellbeing?

Wellbeing is an important word, touted around with little thought to what it means. It became almost ubiquitous in the wake of the pandemic, when everyone suddenly realised how important their wellbeing was. Higher levels of it are associated with lots of lovely things, such as increased life satisfaction, improved mental health, decreased risk of disease (and illness and injury), better immune system functioning and more. Increased wellbeing in the workplace means your employees are not only more productive, but also less prone to taking time off work sick with stress. But what is 'wellbeing'?

Simply put, wellbeing is a state of being comfortable, or healthy, or happy, or all the above. It can be described as seeing life in a positive way and feeling good about yourself and with your life. It is a state of satisfaction.

According to a Gallup study of people across 150 countries, there are five factors that shape our wellbeing: physical, financial, career, social and community.

Meanwhile, the National Wellness Institute promotes six dimensions of wellness: emotional, occupational, physical, social, intellectual and spiritual. The idea is that the more you are taking care of these dimensions, the more satisfied you are with these domains, then the healthier and happier you will feel.

However, before we delve any deeper into the dimensions of wellbeing, I'm going to immediately increase yours by asking you to sit in a chair or lie on the floor, and then relax every single muscle in your body. Not only will the regular practice of this do wonderful things for your stress levels but, if you practise it in bed, it could also have you falling into a deep and relaxing sleep in just a few minutes. Lowering stress and improving sleep are two wellbeing essentials and, therefore, foundational to what comes after.

Hypnotic mental massage

Stress is going to be a theme that runs as a thread throughout the rest of this book. Nothing impacts your wellbeing and resilience, as well as your physical and mental health, quite like stress. Although the word has become so pervasive and all-encompassing that we've lost sight of what it means (more on that in the next chapter), we do know that managing it more effectively isn't just important, it's vital.

Stress management isn't just about controlling your thoughts or your environment. Learning how to relax your body can also help you cope much better with stress. Stress affects your body as you tense your muscles more often than is healthy for you. That tension typically collects in your back, shoulders and neck, but it can affect other areas, too. Tension headaches are often a result of your inability to control stress in a healthy way.

Progressive muscle relaxation is a tool that is taught in most stress management programmes. Some schools of thought advocate deliberately tensing muscle groups one by one, to recognise what tension feels like, before relaxing those muscle groups, again one by one, so that you learn how to let it go. Other schools of thought do away with deliberately tensing the muscles. The idea is we already know they're tense from stress. So, they cut straight to the chase and get you to practise muscle relaxation immediately.

When practised in self-hypnosis, any progressive muscle relaxation technique becomes deeper, more focused and much more relaxing. When undertaken on a regular basis, you are teaching your muscles to let go of tension, which will have numerous benefits for both body and mind. Think of it as a hypnotic, mental massage.

Not only is it a mental massage, but it is also a great tool for getting a good night's sleep. You may or may not have heard of the Military Sleep

Method. It went viral on social media in 2022 and was then picked up by the traditional media. Developed by the US military to help exhausted soldiers fall asleep deeply and quickly wherever they found themselves, it promises that you will do exactly that and within minutes, provided that you practise regularly.

The method itself involves first relaxing all the muscles in your face as completely as you can, then doing the same in your neck, shoulders and arms, before allowing that relaxation to spread through your chest, back and abdomen and then finally moving down into your legs. The final part of the process asks that you clear your mind by holding a relaxing image in your mind and/or by repeating 'don't think' over and over in your head for about ten seconds.

According to the US military, it works on 96 per cent of people who give it a go. In addition, thousands of TikTokers have allegedly used it to good effect.

As an additional benefit, one study showed that progressive muscle relaxation is also good at improving both sleep quality and anxiety in people dealing with Covid-19.

The script is given below, so you can practise it yourself in self-hypnosis, or record it on your smartphone and play it back to yourself. Or scan the QR code on page 8 for a version of it spoken by me.

2. 'Progressive muscle relaxation' script

Make yourself comfortable ... and gently allow your eyes to close ... and as you sit there or lie there ... with your eyes comfortably closed ... I want you to allow every single muscle in your body to become perfectly calm ... perfectly still ... and perfectly relaxed ...

First the muscles in your head and your face ... let them become perfectly calm ... perfectly still ... and perfectly relaxed ... now ... the muscles in your forehead ... and around your eyes ... let them become perfectly calm ... perfectly still ... and perfectly relaxed ... now ... the muscles in your jaw ... let them become perfectly calm ... perfectly still ... and perfectly relaxed ... just allow your whole head and face ... to become perfectly calm ... perfectly still ... and perfectly relaxed ...

And ... that drowsy ... comfortable feeling ... is descending ... down into your neck ... and into your shoulders ... down into your arms ... your hands ... and your fingers ... let your neck muscles relax ... let them become perfectly calm ... perfectly still ... and perfectly relaxed ... now ... the muscles of your shoulders ... let them become perfectly calm ... perfectly still ... and perfectly relaxed ... now ... the muscles of your arms ... and hands ... and fingers ... let them become perfectly calm ... perfectly still ... and perfectly relaxed ... just allow your hands ... arms ... shoulders ... and neck ... to become perfectly calm ... perfectly still ... and perfectly relaxed ... and that wonderful ... comfortable ... drowsy feeling ... is drifting down further still ...

Let your stomach muscles relax ... let them become perfectly calm ... perfectly still ... and perfectly relaxed ... now ... the muscles of your chest ... your body ... and your back ... let them become perfectly calm ... perfectly still ... and perfectly relaxed ... Just allow your whole body ... to become perfectly calm ... perfectly still ... and perfectly relaxed ... and you are feeling ... more and more comfortable ... you are feeling warm and comfortable ... and completely at peace ...

And that feeling of deep comfort is drifting down further still ... first the muscles of your thighs ... let them become perfectly calm ... perfectly still ... and perfectly relaxed ... now ... the muscles of your calves ... let them become perfectly calm ... perfectly still ... and perfectly relaxed ... now ... the muscles of your feet and ankles ... down to your very toes ... let them become perfectly calm ... perfectly still ... and perfectly relaxed ... just allow your legs to become ... perfectly calm ... perfectly still ... and perfectly relaxed ...

Now ... your whole body is at rest ... perfectly calm ... perfectly still ... and perfectly relaxed ... from the top of your head ... all the way down through your body ... down to the tips of your toes ... perfectly calm ... perfectly still ... and perfectly relaxed ... now ...

I want you to think of a peaceful ... tranquil scene ... maybe a place in nature ... such as a beach ... or perhaps a lake ... maybe you're in a forest ... or a park ... perhaps you are somewhere you have visited ... or maybe you are seeing a place that you'd like to visit ... or perhaps this is a place that simply exists in your imagination ... but it is somewhere you feel perfectly calm ... perfectly still ... and perfectly relaxed ...

If you're using it as a method for sleep, don't forget to repeat 'don't think' in your head for about ten seconds at the end of the script.

While on the subject of sleep, do you remember that in Chapter 4, I said that counting down from ten to one can also be practised in bed, but there it might become a tool for getting a good night's sleep rather than a method for going into a trance? Well, here, progressive muscle relaxation isn't just a stressbusting technique, or a method for getting a good night's sleep, or a Covid aid – it can also be another method for going into a state of self-hypnosis. So, now you know two techniques for doing this: counting down from ten to one or progressive muscle relaxation. If you want to go even deeper you can use both together, one after the other. You can do this in any order but I prefer to use progressive muscle relaxation first, followed by counting down from ten to one, and that is what I have done in the recording. I've even included some generic, but positive, beneficial suggestions for you.

Is your body relaxed now? Are you stress- and tension-free? Good, let's get back to those wellbeing factors.

Five ways to wellbeing

Here in the UK, the NHS and various other health organisations and charities promote what is called 'The Five Ways to Wellbeing'. This approach was based on a review of evidence gathered in the government's 2008 *Foresight Project on Mental Capital and Wellbeing*. It wanted to identify five simple, universal actions that anyone could do on an individual level to help themselves feel healthier and happier. The five ways are: connection, activity, taking notice, learning stuff and giving.

Connection

Social relationships are crucial to our mental health and wellbeing. Even the most introverted of us likes to feel connected to someone. If you feel disconnected, reach out. Try talking to people for real, or over the phone, rather than by email or text (shocking, I know!); build a new friendship; rejuvenate a flagging friendship; hold meaningful conversations. One supermarket chain in the Netherlands deliberately opened slow checkout lanes to let people have more social interactions with both the cashiers and each other.

Activity

Physical fitness is also essential. It's associated with lower levels of anxiety and depression (the most common presenting symptoms for therapy) across all age groups. Exercise doesn't have to mean the gym or an exercise class, although it can. It can mean walking to work, or walking at lunchtime, or walking anywhere you can for that matter. It can mean swimming, hiking, playing sport or anything that involves physical exertion.

Taking notice

Mindfulness is both a form of mediation and a form of therapy that helps you to be more present in the moment. Anything that involves you paying more attention to what is going on around you is a mindfulness practice. This heightened awareness enhances your self-understanding, calms you down, allows you to be more objective and even helps you make better life choices. Taking notice is also about savouring as many of life's little joys as you can.

Learning stuff

Learning things is equally good for your mental health. A love of learning is also considered to be a character strength in positive psychology. A character strength is an attribute that, if you possess it and use it correctly, will elevate your mood. Learning doesn't necessarily mean going to college or university or doing an online course; some people love to chat and learn new things about people, while others like to explore and learn new things about their local area. You can also learn new things from reading, using a language app or solving a puzzle.

Giving

It really is better to give than to receive. Kindness is another character strength in positive psychology. Doing something nice for someone allows you to feel good about yourself. Just one kind act a week is enough to significantly improve your mood. And it doesn't have to be a big thing, either: gift giving, cutting a magazine article out for someone whom you think might appreciate it, and saying 'please' and 'thank you' more often all count, but so too do things such as volunteering, getting involved in community projects and giving blood. Being kind boosts your sense of connection to others, and there is plenty of research undertaken in schools, care homes and offices the world over that confirms this.

Lifting Louise

Louise came to see me because she was very stressed indeed. She had returned to work after the birth of her first child, and was finding managing work life, home life, childcare and self-care very difficult. On top of the stress, she had also added the burden of guilt: guilty for not performing as well as she could at work; guilty for being a working mum rather than a stay-at-home mum; guilty for not having enough quality time with her child, her husband or any of her friends; and guilty that she had let her twice-weekly exercise classes (which were very important to her) fall by the wayside. I taught Louise both ten-to-one self-hypnosis and progressive muscle relaxation. I also discussed the five ways to wellbeing with her and we talked about how she might meet these and how they would help her if she did. The script below is based on the one I wrote specifically for her. Hers contained more suggestions that were tailored to her preferences but it has become the basis for a generic template that I have updated time and again over the years and use to help many different people. It is that generic version I am using below. As you get more creative with your self-hypnosis, as you move further towards unconscious competence, please feel free to embellish it and personalise it however you wish.

3. 'Five ways to wellbeing' script

And as you relax in this deep ... hypnotic trance ... I want to speak to your unconscious mind about those five ways to wellbeing ... all the suggestions you hear for your benefit will imprint perfectly on your unconscious mind ... and will activate ... and help you ... when you wish to be helped ... when you wish them to activate ...

You are a social creature ... even the most introverted among us needs to nurture at least one good ... strong social connection ... to another human being ... your social connections are important to you ... they have always been important to you ... sometimes those connections fall by the wayside ... life can get in the way ... work can get in the way ... but here ... in hypnosis ... you can focus on the connections that are important to you ... the ones that could be a little stronger than they currently are ... the ones that have fallen by the wayside ... and you can ... if you wish ... resolve to strengthen those relationships ... perhaps there is someone you would like to call instead of text ... or meet in person rather than call ... maybe you want to talk to people at work in person instead of sending and replying to emails ... you might even be thinking of a person at work whom you like and admire ... and are moved to speak to them in person ... and ask them how they are ... perhaps all of the above ... a kaleidoscope of images ... of social connections ... playing through your mind right now ... and I don't know when you will be moved to act on any of these ideas ... maybe it will be tomorrow ... or the day after ... or next week ... I don't know when exactly you will do this ... but I do know how pleasantly surprised you will be about how good it feels to initiate ... to build ... and to improve these connections ...

And ... as you think about these social connections ... you can also think about your fitness levels ... that innate connection to your own physical body ... are you as connected as you would like to be right now ... are these levels right for you right now ... or do they need improving ... I don't know what being active means to you ... is it a workout in the gym ... or an exercise class ... is it yoga ... or Pilates ... or a mixture of all ... is exercise for you a walk through a park at lunchtime with a friend or work colleague ... I don't know what being active means to you ... but I know it means something to you ... it means something to all of us ... exercise is good for us ... and it is good for you ... and you would like to do more of it, would you not ... perhaps you can see or sense or imagine new ways for you to incorporate daily exercise into your life ... walking ... running ... swimming ... jogging ... working out ... you know what works for you ... and your unconscious mind knows what days and times work best for you ... and I don't know what it will be that you commit to ... will it be few steps a day ... or 10,000 ... will it be the gym once a week or will it be more ... I don't know what it will be that you will commit to ... but I do know you will commit to something ... whatever it is you decide to do ... I want you to see ... or sense ... or imagine yourself doing it now

... committing to it now on a regular basis ... and feeling rather proud of your decision ...

You might also like to make the decision to be more mindful of your surroundings ... more present in each moment ... the past has gone already and the future has yet to arrive ... all we have is here and now ... and so you no longer dwell on the past ... nor worry about the future ... you focus only on the here and now ... and determine to become involved in and absorbed by each passing moment ... and each moment is a notice to take more notice ... of the beauty of your surroundings ... and so from now on you may find yourself slowing down ... savouring life's moments ... a walk in the park ... the laugh of child ... or a friend ... the sun coming through the clouds ... even a queue in a shop is a chance to slow down ... be present ... and savour your surroundings ... take a moment now to savour a few of your life's joys ... allow whatever springs to mind to spring to mind ... and just let yourself become vitally absorbed ... and deeply involved with those images and experiences ...

And these can include moments of learning ... you like to learn new things, do you not ... it could be a course or a workshop ... a new aspect of your job ... perhaps a new language or a musical instrument ... maybe even a book or ... a new route to work through a different part of town ... anywhere and everywhere can be an opportunity to learn something new ... and there is something you are motivated to learn ... either by yourself or from someone else ... see yourself now ... not only becoming vitally absorbed in the day-to-day moments of your life ... but see those moments as opportunities to learn new things ... as prompts to dig deeper ... and investigate further ... and as you dig a little deeper now ... you may be surprised to discover just what it is that you wish to learn ... or to remind yourself of something you have always wanted to learn ... and just take a moment to appreciate how good it will feel when you start to do that ...

Learning is good for your brain ... firing new neurons is good for your wellbeing ... anything you begin to learn ... will change the shape ... and form ... and function of your brain ... and the more you commit to learning something, the better at it you will become ... the more habitual it will be ... just let your mind drift into the future now ... as near or as far into the future as is appropriate for you ... and see yourself at the top of your game ... a master of your chosen skill ...

unconsciously competent ... automatically masterful ... in that skill you chose to learn ... all those weeks ... or all those months ago ...

And maybe you can see yourself getting really good at giving ... there is a saying ... that it is better to give than to receive ... and it is true that being kind makes you feel really good about yourself ... so here in a trance ... those words mean more than you know ... because it is good to give ... good for the person receiving ... but also good for you ... acts of kindness release stress ... and boost happy hormones ... they foster a sense of connection ... and you can give the gift of anything ... a kind word ... a thank you ... a thank-you note ... a moment of your time ... a thoughtful clipping from a magazine ... volunteering ... giving blood and more ... and I wonder what acts of kindness you want to commit to ... I wonder what gifts you want to give ... and I wonder just how easy you are going to find being kind will be ... and how easy to fit into your daily life it is going to become ...

Connecting to others ... becoming more active ... taking more notice of the world around you ... learning new things ... giving more ... perhaps you will only choose two or three of the five ... or maybe you will commit to all of them ... I don't know which ones you will commit to but ... some or all ... I do know whatever ways you commit to ... will enhance your mood ... will increase your wellbeing ... will make you feel more satisfied within yourself and about yourself in every single way ...

Affirmative action

And there you have it, a script that will decrease stress by releasing tension that is also another entry into self-hypnosis plus a good night's sleep all in one, followed by a script that will help increase overall wellbeing.

Because actions speak louder than words, after I had used these hypnotherapy protocols with Louise, I got her to not only practise them regularly in self-hypnosis, but to also write down and commit to the various things she saw herself doing during the hypnosis session and report her progress in the next session. Perhaps you would also like to write down and commit to whatever you became aware of while in the trance state.

Any positive action you commit to will be good for you. As I mentioned previously, nothing impacts your mental health, your wellbeing and your resilience quite like stress.

In the next chapter, the work continues. Not only will I help you bust some more stress, but I will also be busting some myths about stress.

8

Stress and how to handle it

According to the World Health Organization, 'stress can be defined as a state of worry or mental tension caused by a difficult situation. Stress is a natural human response that prompts us to address challenges and threats in our lives. Everyone experiences stress to some degree. The way we respond to stress, however, makes a big difference to our overall wellbeing.'

The last part of that quote is quite important because we've been taught that stress is a bad thing. But there are two types of stress: good and bad.

Eustress

This is positive stress. The 'eu' bit is a prefix (meaning 'good') and refers to the sort of pressure and challenge that we thrive under, or rise to meet and, even, enjoy. Think about the enjoyable pressures of a deadline that you feel in control of, or the enjoyable stress of planning and executing a wedding or a holiday. Some people can take this good form of stress to its limit and go BASE jumping or canyoning. We call these people 'buzz junkies' or 'adrenaline junkies'.

Distress

This refers to stress gone bad and is what we are often referring to when we talk about 'stress' ('di' means 'twice,' or 'twofold', or 'double'). Think of the seemingly insurmountable pressures of work and its attendant projects, the weight of which you feel you are collapsing under, or the wedding where everything seems to contain soap opera levels of drama, or the holiday where the booking is messed up, the flight is delayed, and the resort is a half-finished building site next to a cesspit. Think of that type of honeymoon after that kind of wedding that was an escape from that level of work stress.

But stress isn't a diagnosis in and of itself. You can be anxious and stressed, or angry and stressed, or depressed and stressed (or all of the above and stressed). Stress can be a factor in insomnia and can often be a cause of skin conditions such as psoriasis. Irritable bowel syndrome (IBS) is nearly always stress-related. You can turn to unhealthy coping strategies when you are stressed (think junk food, alcohol and drugs, both prescription and recreational). Chronic work stress even has its own diagnosis: burnout syndrome. This is a purely occupational phenomenon that was not officially recognised until 2019. It is characterised by exhaustion, increased negativity (or cynicism) towards your job or situation and reduced professional efficacy.

Stress: such as small word for something with so many ramifications.

Stress affects both your brain and your body. A little bit of it is good for you and can enhance your wellbeing and resilience. But too much stress can overwhelm you. It can wear you down, physically and mentally.

There is a definition of stress that I borrowed from the Health and Safety Executive (HSE) many years ago (they've changed their definition several times since then – head to their website if you want to see what it is now) and I've mangled it quite a bit over time. It goes like this: 'when the demands or constraints of your situation exceed your ability to cope, then you are at risk of becoming distressed'.

And there are two types of 'I can't cope'. There are the emotional 'I can't copes', where you have got yourself into a bit of a pickle, believing that you can't cope with the things that you can actually cope with once you calm down; and then there are the physical 'I can't copes', where you are just trying to do far too much, or are dealing with far more than you can actually handle, and are doing so on a daily or seemingly never-ending basis. Neither is a good thing.

Sadly, modern life means many of us are dealing with far too much every day of our lives. More than our bodies and minds are designed to cope with. Think of the daily pressures of home management, the hellish commute to and from work, the stresses of your actual working day, plus the pressures of looking after the kids, or parents, or both. Think of the stress of dealing with any customer services department; with the telephone queues and being pushed from department to department. It soon adds up. It soon takes its toll. Weekends and five weeks' holiday per annum are not nearly enough time off to recover, should you get paid holiday at all (if you're a freelancer, for example).*

Distress, you see, puts our central nervous system on red alert and triggers the flight, fight or freeze response.

Simple biology lesson alert

There are two sides to our central nervous system: the sympathetic and the parasympathetic. The sympathetic side controls our flight, fight or freeze responses. It prepares us for physical activity and, when there is a danger, it floods out bodies with chemicals (including adrenaline and cortisol) so that we can either fight our way out of the danger, run for our lives, or root to the spot in the hope that the danger passes us by. The parasympathetic side is known as the rest and digest response. It controls your body during times of rest and relaxation. It's also good at clearing out the adrenaline and cortisol. These chemicals are fairly toxic. They're of great benefit in the short term but quite taxing physically and mentally in the long term. Biologically speaking, we are meant to spend most of our days in rest and digest mode, with fight or flight kicking in only when there is a threat, with a return to rest when the danger has passed. However, modern life is so stressful that we spend too much time with our sympathetic nervous system switched on and not nearly enough time engaging the parasympathetic side.

The good news is that the research is very clear on the matter: hypnotherapy lowers your stress levels by switching on the parasympathetic side of your nervous system.

* Medieval peasants had more time off than the average modern worker. The Church and the land barons knew that if they overworked their serfs then they would either revolt, or die, which really is something to think about the next time you're asked to work through lunch.

Say my name

We think of 'freeze' as the rabbit stuck in the headlights response, which is what it can be, and more besides, as my client Julia discovered. She came to see me because she was stressed and anxious. What's more, when she found herself in situations that she found stressful, she typically went rigid with fear. Her mind would then go blank. She came to see me because she had just quit her very stressful job and was applying for, and being interviewed for, new roles. The problem was that she found interviews very stressful and the more intimidating the interview, the more anxiety she felt. Our first meeting came about shortly after she had had a weird and stressful interview. The interview itself was conducted in a very large room with a very high ceiling. There was one table in the middle of the room, behind which sat the three people who would be interviewing her – two women on either side and a man in the middle. There was a chair in front of the table for her to sit on. The man in the middle of the trio of staff held a clipboard that presumably contained her CV and other information. Already nervous before the interview, Julia's anxiety hit the vaulted roof the moment she stepped into the room. Her high heels echoed as she walked across the parquet floor and sat in the chair.

'Name?' barked the person in the middle from behind his clipboard.

'What?' said Julia, wide-eyed with fear.

'I want to know your name,' he stated with severity.

Julia's brain froze, and her name died on her lips. 'I don't know,' she whispered.

'What do you mean, you don't know your name?' he spat.

Julia fled the room in tears. She was crying further still when she sat in my chair. 'I'm Julia,' she sobbed. 'I've been Julia my whole life. Why couldn't I say my name?'

Stress was why; anxiety was why; her heightened nervous system on overload was why and her fight, flight or freeze mode kicking in rather too well was why.

Anything that destresses you, anything that engages the parasympathetic nervous system, anything that triggers the rest and digest response is going to be good for you: removing yourself from a stressful situation, going for a long walk, breathing in some fresh air, taking a break from work, meditation, yoga, tai chi, you name it. It all helps. Practising self-hypnosis by counting from ten to one and using progressive muscle relaxation on a regular basis will help. Putting stressbusting suggestions into your self-hypnosis sessions will help even more. And to help you with that myself, I am going to take you on a trip to a beach on a nice, sunny day. If indeed you do like beaches and nice, sunny days.

If you don't like beaches, and you want to record a version of this yourself, please substitute it for somewhere else; anywhere you find relaxing: a forest, a lake, a mountain – anywhere. Don't forget to use counting down and/or progressive muscle relaxation before you use the script.

4. 'Standing on a beach: stressbuster' script

You are now deeply relaxed ... deeply relaxed ... and as this sense of relaxation continues to deepen ... I want you to focus on your breathing ... and I want you to breathe in and out through your nose ... breathe in through your nose slowly and deeply ... and breathe out through your nose slowly and deeply ... in and out ... through your nose ... slowly and deeply ... through your nose ... slowly and deeply ... and the sound of your breathing relaxes you ... and it sounds ... just like the ocean sounds ... and it sounds ... just like the sea ...

And ... in hearing the waves ... hearing the sea ... I want you to imagine that you are standing on a beach ... on a beautiful day ... the sun is shining ... there is hardly a cloud in the sky ... the temperature of the air on your skin is ... just perfect ... a slight breeze caresses your face ... and the sand feels so warm and comfortable ... beneath your feet and between your toes ... the beach stretches on into forever in either direction ... it really is such a beautiful day ... and you feel very calm ... very comfortable ... you feel safe and secure ... completely at peace ...

And ... the sound of the ocean ... the roar of the waves ... calls to you ... and so you decide to walk down to the water's edge ... to where the sand meets the sea ... the sea stretching out all the way to the horizon ... the sunlight glinting and reflecting off the rolling waves ... the surf lapping on to the beach ... and you once again become aware of your breathing ... in and out through your nose ... slowly and deeply ... and the rhythm of your breathing matches the sound of the ocean ... or perhaps the sound of your breathing matches the rhythm of the ocean ... either way ... you are breathing in the wonderfully clean ... pure ... fresh sea air ... and you are feeling a very deep level of relaxation ... all the tension is going out of your body ... almost as if that tension is drifting away ... out over the sea ... and over the horizon ...

Now ... your whole being is at rest ... from the top of your head ... to the tips of your toes ... every muscle ... every nerve ... every fibre of your being ... is at rest ... your whole body slows down ... your mind slows down ... deep ... and still ... and so very peaceful ... and now healing forces flow through you ... engaging your parasympathetic nervous system ... enhancing it ... and those healing forces are ... repairing ... replacing ... re-energising ... regenerating ... restoring ... clearing out toxins and ... soothing your mind ... soothing your nerves ... rest and digest ... healing and harmonising ... flowing through you ... repairing ... replacing ... re-energising ... regenerating ... restoring ... rest ... and digest ...

You are breathing in the wonderfully clean ... pure ... fresh ... sea air ... you are breathing in health and wellness ... you are breathing out stress and tension ... you are breathing in peace and calm ... you are breathing out all forms of negativity ... you are breathing in balance and clarity ... and you are breathing out all those stressful situations ... people ... and events ... and as you do so ... you feel a wonderful sense of release ... as easy as breathing in ... and breathing out ... breathing in health and wellness ... breathing out stress and tension ... breathing in peace and calm ... breathing out all forms of negativity ... breathing in balance and clarity ... breathing out all those stressful situations ... people ... and events ... feeling again that wonderful sense of release ... as easy as breathing in ... and breathing out ... breathing in health and wellness ... and peace and calm ... and balance and clarity ... breathing out stress and tension ... breathing out all forms of negativity ... breathing out stressful situations ... people ... and events ... to the sound of the ocean ... to the roar of the waves ... to the surf lapping on to the beach ... breathing in the wonderfully clean ... pure ... fresh ... sea air ...

And as you continue this process ... as easy as breathing in and breathing out ... you feel a sense of balance in your mind ... and a sense of balance in your body ... a sense of balance in your muscles ... your nerves ... and the very fibres of your being ... peace ... and calm ... restored to both body and mind ...

And you can stay here for as long as you wish ... you'll only awaken from the trance ... when all those wonderful ... healing changes ... have begun ... so ... whenever you feel that it is time ... I want you to turn around ... and walk back up the beach ... and bring yourself back to full waking consciousness ... bringing all that health ... wellness ... peace ... calm ... balance ... and clarity ... with you as you do so ...

As always, please feel free to read this script yourself a few times, memorise it as best you can, and replay it in your mind in self-hypnosis. Alternatively, you can record it yourself on your smartphone, or download my version of it using the QR code on page 8.

If you think that the above sounds a little bit like a holiday, it does (or at least it can). I have elaborated on that script for myself and others to make it even more holiday-like on many occasions; a whole two-weeks' worth of images and expressions, from booking the flight to checking in; from lounging on the beach to sultry al fresco evenings and all the way back home again.

Hypno-holidays, also known as mind travel, became very popular during the pandemic, when no one was allowed to holiday anywhere. The idea of holiday by hypnosis is nothing new, however, as other therapists have been providing this service for years. Celebrity hypnotherapist Paul McKenna, for instance, was offering to take people on a vacation in just 20 minutes (in a booth, in a famous UK shopping centre) as far back as 2015.

I wonder where you will go, and I wonder what you will do. Some of you will already be thinking of far-flung beaches or exciting city breaks, while others will be worrying about the flight and the state of the hotel. There's a fine line between caution and catastrophising, and we are very good at crossing it. The next chapter, however, is all about breaking those negative thought cycles.

9

Stop negative thinking

Have you ever wondered why you're so negative? Well, wonder no more. Because you can't help it. None of us can. It's biological, it's hardwired into all of us. Our brains aren't built for happiness, they're built for survival. Once upon a time, this was strictly necessary.

Our brains haven't evolved that much over the millennia. If you go back in time to when we were all living in hunter-gatherer tribes, our brains and our bodies were pretty much the same then as they are now. And back then we needed a brain that was very much disaster aware.

As hunter-gatherers, when you broke camp, you went out to hunt and gather. When you returned, it might have been nice to talk about what a lovely day you'd just had picking berries or hunting gazelle but, really, you needed to talk about the dangers. You needed to talk about the immediate dangers: don't go that way (quicksand!), and don't go that way (sabre-tooth tigers!). That kind of thing. But you also needed to talk about the long-term dangers: hard winters looking likely, herds moving on early, and so on. Because if you didn't talk about and prepare for these dangers, your tribe would die out. It would become extinct.

Fast-forward to today and metaphorically speaking, we still break camp in the morning. We are still hunting and gathering and, when we return at the end of the day, our survivalist brains are still bringing home the dangers. Only, it's not quicksand and sabre-tooth tigers, or early winters and vanishing food stocks; but non-life-threatening stuff such as traffic jams, horrible conversations, poor performance reviews, the cost-of-living crisis, various interpersonal difficulties and more. Challenging yes, often unpleasant, but not something to let consume us.

In their book *The Power of Bad*, the authors and psychologists John Tierney and Roy F. Baumeister argue that it takes four positive things to overcome one negative thing.

Just because this bias towards negativity is a biological imperative, it doesn't mean it can't be overcome, it doesn't mean you can't build a habit whereby you stop negative thinking. It just takes effort (and an average of 66 days). Thanks to neuroplasticity, you can hardwire a happier brain. And hypnotherapy can help. So too can throwing things at people.

Paper, ping-pong balls and Nerf guns

Carlos came to see me as he was suffering from work-related stress. He was also a self-described 'super-catastrophiser' and was quite aware that his doom-mongering brain was a big factor in his stress management (or lack thereof). It didn't help that he worked in financial risk management. His negative thinking was quite something. Several sessions in and, quite often, it was all that he brought into the room. We were both quite frustrated by this, but in a jovial fashion.

'You should throw the book at me,' he said after one such swerve into Negative Nellie Land.

'Oh, I'd like to throw something at you,' I replied in jest. Thirty seconds later, when he voiced yet another baseless worst-case-scenario thought, I scrunched a sheet of A4 paper up into a ball and lobbed it at him. He laughed.

'That might work,' he said.

Although I did this on impulse, the technique itself was not without precedent. One way to distract your negative thoughts is via the rubber band 'snap'. The idea is to wear a rubber band around your wrist (or a wristband deliberately fashioned for such a purpose) and then flick it every time you become aware of a negative thought. It can take a while to break that neural pathway so you may be flicking away for many days, weeks or even months, but it does work well. By the end of my session with Carlos, there were many balled-up pieces of paper on the floor and we both lamented that his newfound awareness was going to be very detrimental to trees. At the next session, Carlos came in with a big tub of ping-pong balls for me to throw at him, which I did. Slowly but steadily, the number of balls that needed to be thrown (and retrieved) reduced over time.

Towards the end of our work together, Carlos gave me an article he had cut out from a magazine. 'You're going to love this,' he said. The article was a piece about a therapist who shot his patients with a Nerf gun every time they said something bad about themselves. Shooting people with foam darts is both a valid and effective CBT technique. But with Carlos (and others), I backed up the ping-pong balls with the following hypnotherapy script.

5. 'Stop negative thinking' script

I want to speak to your unconscious mind about your negative thinking ... and I wonder if you might consider ... what happens when ... you imagine yourself ... not thinking negatively ... perhaps you have already considered it ... and because you have already considered it ... you find yourself ready to change ... because your unconscious mind ... has already decided ... that you are ready for change ...

From now on ... you are going to be very consciously aware of your negative thoughts ... and whenever you notice a negative thought entering your mind ... you are going to shout out STOP ... in a very loud but internal voice ... you are going to shout out STOP ... and at the same time ... you are going to see ... or sense ... or imagine ... a bright red light flashing as a warning ... and if not a bright red light ... then you will hear ... or sense ... or imagine ... a loud alarm going off ... and if not that ... then perhaps you will feel ... or sense ... or imagine a rubber band around your wrist being flicked ... and feel a short ... sharp ... shock of awareness ... perhaps you will even imagine a combination of all three ... either way ... you will immediately resolve to stop negative thinking ... and at the same time ... you will remember a peaceful ... tranquil scene ... something that makes you smile ...

And I want you to know that as soon as you hear yourself criticise yourself ... either internally or externally ... as soon as a negative thought about yourself ... enters your mind ... you are going to instantly

... and immediately ... turn it into a humorous voice ... a silly voice ... a cartoon voice ... maybe you will speed that voice up ... or slow that voice down ... maybe you will use the voice of a cartoon character ... or comedian ... and as soon as you have altered that voice ... as soon as you have made it silly ... you will immediately replace that critical thought with something kind ... you will immediately say something kind ... and caring ... about yourself ...

Is there a part of you that wants to stop thinking so negatively ... there is ... is there not ... is there a part of you that wants to learn how to do this ... really quickly ... there is ... isn't there ...

And so ... you are going to get very good ... at reducing your negative thinking ... and as the days ... and the weeks ... and the months go by ... and you become increasingly competent at reducing negative thoughts ... you will find that you have reduced those negative thoughts ... down to almost nothing at all ... almost nothing at all ... and you are going to find that your mind has increasingly defaulted to positive thoughts ... peaceful thoughts ... and kind thoughts about yourself ... and perhaps ... you might like to commit to thinking this way ... as often as possible ... for as long as possible ... until this becomes habitual ... and automatic for you ...

If you are going to record this script for yourself, it will be very helpful if you repeat it (feel free to ad-lib) at least three times before waking yourself up.

Stop negative images

Some people think less in negative thoughts about themselves and the situations they are in and more in terms of images, sometimes very vivid worst-case-scenario scenes. Like a disaster movie in their head. And these can be stopped in a very similar way to the above. So, if you want to break out your smartphone and record a script like the above but to cater for vivid imagery instead, you can adapt the following:

Perish the thought

Whenever a negative image enters your mind, first focus on it and make it very clear and vivid, then shrink it down, allow it to become smaller and smaller, then turn down the brightness and make the image hazier and less distinct. Notice how you feel about it. Notice how your feelings towards it have changed, even. Then push that image further and further away, pushing it into the distance, allowing it to become small, indistinct, a little dot on the horizon and then let it disappear over that horizon. And then, in the distance, coming over the same horizon, allow yourself to see a new, pleasant, happy, peaceful image; an image that you know is going to make you smile. An image that you know will produce feelings of confidence and positivity. Bring that image closer and closer, allow it to grow brighter, clearer and more vivid. When it gets really close to you, step into that image and soak up all the feelings of positivity and confidence. If you are going to record this, repetition is key, so repeat these suggestions at least three times.

Accentuate the positive

This isn't just the name of a song originally sung by Bing Crosby and The Andrews Sisters, it is also another good habit to build, and one where you simply focus on the positive. It doesn't mean that you ignore the negative or pretend it isn't there, and it certainly doesn't mean that you can't talk about the challenges you face (bottling things up and ignoring them doesn't do anyone any good) but, instead of focusing on the negative, you can choose to accentuate the positive. As mentioned earlier, the famous hypnotherapist Milton Erickson, who was colour blind, tone-deaf, had dyslexia and later contracted polio, was a firm believer in doing so.

Also known as looking on the bright side, it does involve thinking a little outside the box. So, for instance, instead of bemoaning the accident that has you in traction for the next six weeks, you could say you've been given the time to read some good books. Or let's say you get fired from your job suddenly, instead of focusing on the worst-case scenario or swearing vengeance against the company that got rid of you, you could see it as a chance to update your CV, reflect on your skill set and point yourself in another direction.

So, with that in mind, here is a very short script on emphasising the positive. Please feel free to add it to the 'Stop negative thinking' script (*see* pp. 87–88) or, indeed, any other script you see fit, or any hypnotherapy session of your own that you develop.

6. 'Accentuate the positive' script

I want you to know that you are in control of your mind ... always ... you are in control of your mind ... and because you are in control of your mind ... from now on ... you will choose to emphasise the positive as much as possible ... in the past ... you may have emphasised the negative ... and minimised the positive ... but ... from now on ... you choose to reverse this tendency ... and instead ... you will emphasise the positive ... and minimise the negative ... you will emphasise the positive ... and minimise the negative ...

There is a saying ... that every cloud has a silver lining ... it is a bit of a cliché but it's true ... but it is also true that a cliché only becomes a cliché because it is true ... and meaningful ... relevant ... and revealing ... and it is also true ... that something good can often be found in most bad situations ... not all ... but most ... and from now on ... your mind will focus on the good in a bad situation ... and you are going to get really good at finding the good in a bad situation ... it doesn't mean that you can ignore the bad ... or that you will even want to ... but you can minimise it ... reduce it ... and favour the positive ... while reflecting on ... and learning from the bad ...

Failure is an opportunity to learn ... convalescence is an opportunity to rest ... the end of a relationship is a chance to rediscover yourself ... and the end of a job ... is the chance to discover what else is out there ...

And best of all ... from now on ... you will actively choose ... for the benefit of your wellbeing ... to emphasise the positive ... and minimise the negative ...

And the more you practise, the better you will get ... and the better you get ... the more you will want to practise ... until one day ... and I don't know when exactly ... but one day ... soon ... emphasising the positive ... accentuating the positive ... is going to be easy for you ... effortless for you ... habitual for you ...

And while staying with the topic of emphasising the positive, in the next chapter we are going to delve a little deeper into positive psychology.

10

The power of positive psychology

I've already mentioned positive psychology once or twice. Whereas most forms of psychotherapy are concerned with your mental illnesses and how to make you better (always a good thing), with the implicit understanding that your mental health and wellbeing will improve, positive psychology focuses only on your mental wellness. It is the study of human happiness. It involves establishing what makes life worth living. Positive psychology aims to improve your quality of life and enhance your wellbeing.

It entered the psychological mainstream in 1998 when a psychologist called Martin Seligman chose it as the theme for his term as president of the American Psychological Association.

Like hypnotherapy, positive psychology can complement traditional areas of psychology and, like both hypnotherapy and rational emotive behaviour therapy (REBT), positive psychology can also be used as a form of coaching and therapy and – when used on life in general – can give you a great way of looking at things in a happier, calmer and more productive way.

There is a misconception that with positive psychology you are only supposed to focus on the positive, while totally discounting the negative.

Its detractors have labelled this 'toxic positivity'. That is not how it is meant to be used. If someone, either in a professional or a personal context, is invalidating your experience while telling you to look on the bright side, they are using positive psychology wrongly. There is a whole world of difference between telling yourself everything is great while everything around you is falling apart, and telling yourself that while everything is falling apart, you will do your best to draw something positive from the experience.

As mentioned in Chapter 5, the self-improvement psychotherapist Émile Coué was the originator of the optimistic self-help mantra, 'every day in every way, I'm getting better and better'.

Studies show that positive affirmations do indeed improve wellbeing but, in my experience, they only work when used correctly. So, 'every day in every way, I'm getting better and better' works only if every day in every way, you are indeed getting better and better (even if only a little bit). If you're not, then the affirmation is simply plastering over the cracks. So, affirmations work best when used alongside affirmative action and, if things are very challenging indeed, other forms of therapy to help you work on your stuff. To my mind, positivity only becomes toxic when it's either misused accidentally or misunderstood entirely or, horror of horrors, deliberately used to negate your challenges and your feelings about them.

Positive psychology has a lot to say about resilience and how to handle tough and challenging situations with more fortitude and I will be touching on these and other subjects in the next section. But for now, I want to delve a little deeper into two topics mentioned at the beginning of this section, namely gratitude and kindness. Gratitude first, because bringing this into your life will work wonders.

When you express gratitude on a regular basis, it can increase happiness, elevate mood, improve life satisfaction levels, make you less materialistic and less likely to experience burnout, improve sleep, decrease fatigue, increase resilience, improve your physical health, reduce bodily inflammation and encourage the development of patience, humility and wisdom. Blimey!

One such study, involving more than 1300 participants, found that gratitude exercises not only increased subjective happiness but also decreased depressive symptoms. It has even been shown that a course of positive psychology for treating depression can be as just as effective as a course of CBT for depression.

I ran a positive psychology group at the Priory Hospital Bristol for seven years and gratitude was an essential component of every session. In any group setting (psychotherapeutic, professional, educational, social care and so on), gratitude increases prosocial behaviours, strengthens relationships, improves social cohesion, makes you feel more connected to others and (at work) can increase employee effectiveness. And it all starts with one simple exercise.

Three things: a gratitude journal

Keeping a journal is a great way to look after your mental health. Practically every form of therapy advocates keeping one. Different therapies use it in different ways. Some use it to explore your emotions or to understand them better, while others encourage you to actively challenge your more dysfunctional thoughts through journaling. A positive psychology diary would employ exercises that encourage mood improvement. In that respect, one of the best things you can do is to write down three things you are grateful for, several days a week. But don't write them down as a bullet-point list. The gratitude is in the detail and so, for each point, sketch out a few words that explain why you are grateful for that thing and then reflect for a few moments on what you have written. So, a typical journal entry could look like this:

Tuesday

1. The spring: I love the spring. I love the way the weather shifts, the sun comes out and things begin to bloom. In the park my home is built in, snowdrops and crocuses bloom and plants begin to bud. It's a lovely sight and a lovely feeling. In fact, I am looking at the snowdrops and crocuses on a bright sunny spring right now as I write this entry.
2. My dog: I love dogs and consider them essential to my wellbeing. I couldn't imagine my home without one. My dog makes me laugh, makes me smile, gives me a warm fuzzy glow and is always pleased to see me. She lifts me up whenever I am feeling low, and all dogs can teach you the true meaning of unconditional love. Today my dog learned a new trick and I am very proud.

3. Books: I love reading. I was a very good reader from a young age. I also consider reading very good for my mental health. I love fiction drawn from a variety of genres and non-fiction on a wide variety of subjects. You can lose yourself in a really good book, find yourself in a really good book and learn some amazing things from a really good book.

I consider a sense of gratitude an essential component of my own wellbeing and I practise this exercise almost daily. I have a smart speaker that has been programmed with a reminder. Every night at 8.00 p.m., Alexa tells me to write down three things that I am grateful for and, every night at 8.00 p.m. (if I am there), I do indeed write those things down. However, you need to use this exercise judiciously. If you overdo it, or use it as a form of virtue signalling, or as a way of appearing better than others, or holier-than-thou, gratitude (or ingratitude) can lead to self-importance, arrogance, vanity, a sense of entitlement and a need for admiration and approval. As with most things in life, it's not what you use but how you use it that matters.

It certainly helps my clients, especially when they present with depression.

The best thing about it was...

Geraldine was referred to me by her psychiatrist, specifically for REBT for depression. However, when I discussed how I worked, she was also interested in both hypnotherapy and positive psychology. Because of her mood disorder, Geraldine hated pretty much everything, including her job, her singledom, dating apps, bad dates, good dates with people she wasn't really into, her friends, her current circumstances, the city she was living in and more. She was also a constant cavalcade of calamity. 'My car caught fire and is a write-off,' she said during one session; 'My laptop died,' she said in the next; 'I'm being made redundant because they don't like me,' she said in the session after that. This was quickly followed by, 'My washing machine broke and flooded my flat.' Week after week, calamity after calamity. Even after we made some improvements to her mood with REBT and hypnotherapy, the calamities continued. And so, I introduced the gratitude journal exercise above and the hypnotherapy script below. I used this script with her more than a few times, changing the content of the gratitude reflections each time. When we brought therapy to a close and reflected on all that she had learned, Geraldine enthused about not only the hypnotherapy, but also the gratitude hypnotherapy and the journal entries that it had been based on.

7. 'Gratitude: engaging the senses' script

As you continue to relax ... I want you to focus on one thing that you are really grateful for ... it can be anything ... anything at all ... a person ... a moment in time ... an act of kindness ... an accomplishment ... anything at all ... and as you focus on that thing ... I want you to locate that sense of gratitude in your body ... is it in your heart ... or your mind ... or your stomach ... wherever it is ... allow that sense of gratitude to grow ... and grow ... allow it to radiate out from that place ... until it encompasses all of you ... until you feel enveloped by ... cocooned by ... gratitude ... and then ...

I want you to engage your senses ... first the sense of touch ... allow yourself to think of ... to be reminded of three things you enjoy touching ... or caressing ... or stroking ... they could be anything ... a fabric ... a pet ... a sandy beach ... anything at all ... just let your mind wander across three things you can touch ... that you are grateful for ... and link that feeling to the gratitude that encompasses your body ... and allow that feeling to grow ... and then ...

I want you to engage with your sense of hearing ... allow yourself to think of ... be reminded of three things you enjoy hearing ... they could be anything ... the sound of the ocean ... a favourite song ... the voice of someone you love ... just let your mind wander across three things you can hear ... that you are grateful for ... and link that feeling to the gratitude that encompasses your body ... and allow that feeling to grow ... and then ...

I want you to engage with your sense of sight ... allow yourself to think of ... be reminded of three things you enjoy seeing ... they could be anything ... the colour of the sky on a perfect day ... a favourite place in nature ... the face of someone you care about ... just let your mind wander across three things you can see ... that you are grateful for ... and link that feeling to the gratitude that encompasses your body ... and allow that feeling to grow ... and then ...

Now ... I want you to engage with your sense of smell ... allow yourself to think of ... be reminded of three things you enjoy the scents and aromas of ... they could be anything ... your favourite food ... your favourite fabric softener ... your favourite perfume or aftershave ... just let your mind wander across three things you can smell ... that you are grateful for ... and link that feeling to the gratitude that encompasses your body ... and allow that feeling to grow ... and then ...

Now ... I want you to engage with your sense of taste ... allow yourself to think of ... be reminded of three things you enjoy tasting ... they could be anything ... your favourite dinner ... your favourite drink ... perhaps it can be something savoury or perhaps something sweet ... just let your mind wander across three things you can taste ... that you are grateful for ... and link that feeling to the gratitude that encompasses your body ... and allow that feeling to grow ... and then ...

And you might consider ... what happens when you imagine yourself already transformed ... by gratitude ... gratitude for things you can touch ... hear ... see ... smell ... and taste ... and that feeling of gratitude ... can only be enhanced ... each time you engage the senses ... each time you touch something pleasing ... each time you hear something soothing ... each time you see something wonderful ... or smell something delightful ... each time you taste something delicious ... so that ... this sense of gratitude is enhanced ... over the days ... and the weeks ... and the months to come ... gratitude for everything you touch ... hear ... see ... smell ... and taste ... and then ...

Cool to be kind

Research has shown that kindness can help alleviate the symptoms of stress, including anxiety and depression. It is a great antidote to loneliness, improves a sense of connection to others, and fosters a sense of community and belonging. It distracts you from your problems and woes and, overall, provides you with a big burst of joy. Doing something nice for someone obviously makes them feel good but it makes you feel even better. It triggers the release of your happy hormones. Being kind, then, is an affirmative act of self-care. One big study, itself a meta-analysis of more than 200 kindness studies involving nearly 200,000 people, found that kindness positively contributes to many aspects of wellbeing.

From care homes to workplaces, when asked to initiate random acts of kindness, the results have been nothing but positive. The elderly in care homes have felt less lonely and more connected to their fellow residents; schools have improved both mood and results, while lessening disruptive behaviour; and workplaces the world over have improved wellbeing and productivity, while increasing social cohesion. In most of these studies, the acts of kindness that participants were asked to partake in were selected for their ease and affordability and included things such as:

- Saying please and thank you more often.
- Cutting magazine articles out and giving them to people whom you think would like to read them.
- Buying someone a thank-you card.
- Giving a gift token.
- Not just recommending a book to a reader, but giving them a copy of the book.
- Buying someone a cup of coffee.
- Bringing in treats to share.
- Paying someone a thoughtful and meaningful compliment.
- Doing someone a favour and more.

Other studies broadened the scope a little and asked people to give blood, donate or volunteer to charity, participate in local community projects, do chores and get the shopping in for someone in your neighbourhood that has need, and so on.

And so, I will end this chapter with a hypnotherapy script that builds on your own innate kindness, a topic introduced in the 'Five ways to well-being' script (*see* pp. 73–76).

8. 'The gift of giving' script

And as you rest there ... deeply relaxed ... deeply in a state of trance ... I want you to reflect on kindness ... and what it means to you ... and you may remember someone being kind to you ... and you may remember how that made you feel ... and you may remember being kind to someone ... and you may remember how that made you feel ... remember the kindest thing someone has ever done for you ... and just experience that moment now as it was then ... perhaps it was something they did ... or something they said ... maybe it was someone you know ... or maybe a complete stranger stopping to help for a moment ... maybe it was a big thing ... maybe a small thing ... but just take a moment and relive those feelings that you had then ... and then ... when you are ready ... remember the kindest thing you have ever done for someone else ... go back in time ... to a memory of a kindness you showed to someone else ... and just experience that moment as it was then ... again ... it could be something you did ... or something you said ... it could be for someone you know or a complete stranger ... it could be a small act of kindness ... or a larger act ... but just take a moment and relive those feelings that you had then ... and then ... when you are ready ... let that feeling grow ... bathe in that warm and happy glow of kindness ... that feeling of connection to other people ... that little burst of joy that starts in the heart ... the mind ... or the soul ... and then radiates outward across your whole being ... and then reflect ... on what kindness means to you ... and how you can be more kind in this world ... now ... I don't know what kindness means to you ... maybe it's saying please and thank you more often ... holding doors open more often ... letting people in and out in traffic jams more often ... paying people compliments more often ... sending thank-you notes and gifts of appreciation more often ... maybe all of the above ... any and all interactions are an opportunity for a kind word ... or kind deed ... and I don't know what exactly it is you will do ... or for whom ... or how often ... but I do know ... that when you do something kind for someone then you feel really good about yourself ... when you do something good ... then you feel more happy ... more connected ... more satisfied with your life ... more appreciative of what you have ... and who you have around you ... whatever it is that you decide to do ... you can notice that not only you but all those people around you are benefitting from your new behaviour ... this unconscious habit of being kind ...

Now you can record one script, the other script, or record them both together. I've included them both together for you in my recordings (see the QR code on page 8). However, increasing your wellbeing isn't just about building good habits. As you will find out in the next chapter, it's also about breaking bad ones.

11

Breaking bad habits

If you are problem drinking (misusing alcohol on a regular basis), this is not the chapter for you. If you have a very unhealthy relationship with food, or think you might have an eating disorder then, similarly, this is not the chapter for you. However, if you think that your relationship with food and/or alcohol is little more than a bad habit that needs nipping in the bud then this is indeed the chapter for you.*

As you have learned elsewhere, we are a collection of habits, patterns of information stored in the unconscious mind; we are what we repeatedly do. If you repeatedly drink more than the recommended amount of units per week (or, even, per night), then that is a habit you have built; if you always choose burgers and pizzas over chicken and salads then unhealthy food is a habit for you, and if you say you really do want to go to the gym but come home each night and plonk your backside down on the sofa, then plonking is a habit for you.

Every single habit, both good and bad, starts with a psychological pattern called a 'habit loop'. This loop is made up of three parts. First, there is the cue or trigger, the thing that tells your brain to go on to autopilot and let the behaviour unfold; then there's the routine or the behavioural element itself (the habit); and, finally, we have the reward – something you like, something you get out of it, something that your brain will latch on to so that it will remember the loop in the future.

* Substance misuse and eating disorders need the help of a trained, specialist professional.

As soon as any behaviour becomes habitual, it becomes automatic (66 days on average). And as soon as that happens, your brain works less. This is advantageous, in that it allows you to focus on other things (think about talking to your friend hands-free while parking the car, that sort of thing) but also disadvantageous as you stop questioning why you are doing it.

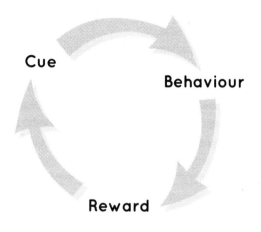

Cue

Behaviour

Reward

THE HABIT LOOP

The good news is that bad habit loops can be broken, new habit loops can be built, and hypnotherapy can help; in fact, it's something hypnotherapy is incredibly good at doing. But it's not a magic wand, and it will also take effort and commitment on your part. And that is easier said than done, mainly due to one of the most pernicious obstacles in your healthy habits path.

Advertising

Weight control is a lot harder than people (including some therapists) think. Diets don't work. Or they do, but only while you are on them. The only way to healthy weight control is through a lifetime plan of healthy eating and regular exercise. The biggest problem to the achievement of that is advertising. In magazines, on billboards and on television, gorgeous, sumptuous food is literally thrust down our throats, only the people eating all the food are actors and models, so they always look beautiful and svelte.

And it's the same with alcohol. Adverts of happy people having fun abound, with the words 'drink responsibly' appearing somewhere on them in teeny-tiny letters. We all know how bad too much booze is – for your organs but also your weight and body fat levels – but we live in a world where alcohol is legal and it is socially acceptable to drink lots of it. 'Go on,' you say to friends, 'just one, it's my birthday-slash-engagement-slash-wedding-slash-whatever.' And boom, you consume additional calories that over time add up to weight gain.

And so, this chapter will help you to stop eating fattening foods, limit your drinking and get you off the sofa and out into whatever form of exercise you consider right for you. I'll even help you fight the advertising and well-meaning friends as best I can.

The very first thing you will need to do is write down all the reasons why it's good for you to eat healthily, drink responsibly and exercise regularly.

Lisa's list

Lisa came to see me because she wanted to lose weight. At the time she presented to me, she ate far too many takeaway meals and snacked far too often on crisps and chocolate. She wanted to go down three dress sizes and had even brought in a picture of her at her ideal size and weight in a dress she loved.*

When I asked her why giving up these things would be good for her, she said, 'Because I don't want to be fat, I don't want to spend money I can't afford on junk food and I don't want to ruin my health.' These are good reasons, it's true, but Lisa was telling me what she didn't want, not what she did want, and so her list wasn't going to help motivate her. With a little bit of prompting, she changed her list to this:

- **I want to be size 12**
  I love being this size, it's good for my body shape, it's perfect for my height, most of my best clothes are this size and I will feel good about myself.†

---

* Having a picture of yourself at your ideal weight and size somewhere handy is a powerful visual motivator.

† Of course, what makes Lisa feel good is not necessarily the same for everyone – this is just an example of a size that is naturally healthy for one person.

- I will save money

  I can update my wardrobe and go to nice places with friends; even saving for a holiday will be easier and I can probably upgrade the type of holiday I usually go for.

- I will be healthier

  My cardiovascular system will improve, my immune system will improve, my complexion will improve. I will be motivated to exercise more and will be happy knowing I'm doing all I can to safeguard my health.

And that is what we mean by a 'list'. It's not a single-word list of things you don't want, it is a detailed list of all the things you do want, with very clear explanations underneath of why these are good things for you specifically. Having this list to hand is really going to help you stay the course and ignore advertising's temptations. And it starts with what you are eating.

9. 'Eating healthily' script

You are in control of your eating habits ... you are in control of what you choose to eat ... you are in control of what you eat ... you stop eating ... gross ... fattening food ... you stop eating stomach-heavy unhealthy food ... you stop eating sickly ... sugary food ... you have no desire to consume gross ... fattening ... heavy ... sugary ... unhealthy food ...

You stop eating chocolate ... you stop eating cake ... you stop eating burgers and chips ... you stop eating fried chicken ... you stop eating takeaways ... you have no desire to consume takeaway food ... no desire to consume fried chicken ... no desire to consume ... burgers and chips ... no desire to consume cake ... no desire to consume chocolate in any form at all ...

I want you to think of an image ... of you at your ideal weight and size ... in your favourite clothes ... perhaps an actual photo springs to mind ... maybe a series of images ... perhaps just an image of you that exists in your mind ... one of you at your ideal weight ... and your ideal size ... in your favourite clothes ... and you can see how happy you look ... there is a smile on your lips ... and in your eyes ... your complexion is healthy ... happy ... glowing ... and you keep this image firmly in your mind ... as inspiration ... inspiration to ...

Stop eating chocolate ... you stop eating cake ... you stop eating burgers and chips ... you stop eating fried chicken ... you stop eating takeaways ... you have no desire to consume takeaway food ... no desire to consume fried chicken ... no desire to consume ... burgers and chips ... no desire to consume cake ... no desire to consume chocolate in any form at all ...

And should anyone or anything ... ever try to tempt you ... with anything ... gross ... fattening ... heavy ... sweet ... sugary ... you know your own mind ... you already know the answer ... you will say no ... you want to say no ... you will be so pleased and proud to say no ... I don't want that ... and each time you say that your determination ... will be reinforced ... you are learning to love your body ... to protect your body ... treating it with kindness and respect ... saying no to unhealthy food ... is kindness and respect ...

From now on ... you are building ... reinforcing ... strengthening ... a healthy eating habit ... a healthy way of life ... lighter ... healthier ... menu options appeal to you ... healthy menu options tantalise your tastebuds ... healthy menu options ... satisfy you because they are in line with your goals ... and you also choose healthy snacks ... fresh fruit ... nuts ... whatever is healthy to you ... you prepare your own meals when you have time ... quick ... easy ... healthy meals ... meals that tempt your tastebuds ... delicious ... healthy food ... food that you know is good for you ... food that nourishes your body ... nourishes your soul ...

From now on ... you are building ... reinforcing ... strengthening ... a more healthy eating habit ... a more healthy way of life ... healthy menu options appeal to you ... healthy menu options tantalise your tastebuds ... healthy menu options ... satisfy you because they are in line with your goals ... and you also choose healthy snacks ... fresh fruit ... nuts ... whatever is healthy to you ... you prepare your own meals when you have time ... quick ... easy ... healthy meals ... meals that tempt your tastebuds ... delicious ... healthy food ... food that you know is good for you ... food that nourishes your body ... nourishes your soul ...

Someone once told me that old habits don't die hard ... and they were right ... they don't die at all ... but they do get replaced ... by new habits ... better habits ... habits that ... over time ... become stronger ... and more ingrained ... and it can be easy ... and effortless ... to replace an old habit with a new one ... and stay the course until that habit is ingrained ... and you will stay the course ... and you will replace your unhealthy food ... with healthy options ... will you not ...

Obviously, the above script is a little generic, though it will work. If you are recording your own script, please feel free to insert all the unhealthy foods you wish to eliminate from your diet if they've become a problem. I've said it before, and I'll say it again (you'll find out why in just a moment), but it's worth repeating the suggestions a good three times for maximum effect.

And after the food comes the drinking. If you want to cut down on your drinking, that is.

Drinking responsibly

The following script is based upon an observation of mine. Do you know the expression, 'Three is the magic number?' Well, three is indeed a significant number in religion, spirituality and magic. The philosopher Pythagoras considered it deeply significant. In fact, the Ancient Greeks thought it the number of harmony, wisdom and understanding. It also represents beginnings, middles and ends, and our brains like narrative structure; they find things grouped in threes more appealing and easier to remember.

It's why hypnotherapy scripts work so well when repeated three times, especially when breaking bad habits or building good ones. It's also the number of drinks at which I can sensibly stop. Up to three is my limit as, after that, I know that drink number four will not be the last drink of the night or session.

This observation of mine has been echoed by many. People who don't want to abstain from drinking but just get it under control always say 'two or three' when asked by me at what point they wish to stop. And they wish it for the same reason as I do: drink number four is the point of no return. Drink number four often leads to many more, which then lends itself to waking up in the morning with a patchy memory at best, wondering why you did it and, also, possibly worrying about what you did.[*]

And so, I developed the script on the next page, not only for myself, but also for all those who want to avoid those kinds of mornings. For all those who want to make it home unscathed. Again, the script is generic, but you can substitute the term 'alcoholic drink' with the drink or drinks you wish to reduce.

---

[*] This is inevitably followed by the question, 'Where the hell am I?'

10. 'No more than three' script

You are in control of your drinking ... always ... you are in control of your drinking ... and you are going to feel so good ... to be in control of your drinking ...

You have decided ... to drink no more than three alcoholic drinks in any one go ... in any one session ... no more than three ... and maybe not even that ... now I don't know ... if you will decide to drink no alcohol at all on occasion ... and I don't know if you will stop at just the one drink on any particular occasion ... and I don't know if you will stop at two drinks on any particular occasion ... but I do know that you will definitely stop at three ... because you know that is your limit ... that is you in control ... and you are in control ... are you not ...

Three is your limit ... maybe even two ... perhaps one ... and maybe even none at all ... maybe soft drinks only ... whatever you are comfortable with at the time ... but you are in control ... and three is your limit ... three is the magic number ... three is the perfect number ... the number of harmony ... wisdom ... and understanding ... and so stopping at three represents you in harmony ... according to your wisdom ... with your complete understanding ... and so ... you have no desire to drink more than three alcoholic drinks on any one occasion ... you have no desire to drink more than three alcoholic drinks in one go ... you have no desire to drink any more than three alcoholic drinks at any given time ever again ...

Of course ... in the past ... you used to drink more than three ... in the past ... you would sail right past three ... because you did not have that harmony ... and you did not have that wisdom ... and you did not have that understanding ... and you found it difficult to stop because ... as you know ... most people find it difficult to stop ... when they have drunk more than three ... but also ... in the past ... you found it difficult to stop ... because your unconscious mind didn't know ... didn't understand ... that you wanted to stop at three ... it was basing your habits on all your previous nights out ... on that lack of harmony ... . that lack of wisdom ... that lack of understanding ... but here ... in hypnosis ... your unconscious mind fully understands ... fully accepts ... that you want to stop at three ... and your unconscious mind ... the most harmonious ... the most wise ... and the most understanding part of you ... can communicate that fact to every single part of you ... so that every single part of you understands ... that you will stop at three ... perhaps even two on occasion ... and sometimes one ... or none ... you decide on the night ... but you are in control ... and you have no desire to drink more than three ... you are learning to love your body ... to protect your body ... treating it with kindness and respect ... and stopping at three ... is kindness and respect ...

Because three is the magic number and because it takes a good three weeks minimum to build a new habit, the following script can help as a booster.

11. 'Staying focused' script

Your mind is strong ... you are focused ... you are determined ... you stick to your goals ... you remind yourself of all the reasons your goals are good goals for you ... people admire your determination to succeed ... and because you are focused on success ... advertising for food and drink means nothing to you ... carefully edited pictures and television adverts of unhealthy food will not tempt you ... will not deter you from your goals ... people saying ... go on ... just this once ... will not break your willpower ... if you decide to eat something or drink something ... it is because you decided to do it ... but ... you stick to your guns ... you stick to your goals ... you keep your eyes on the prize ... nothing ... and no one ... can force you ... no one and nothing ... can persuade you ... your mind is strong ... you are focused ... you are determined ... people admire your willpower ... your determination to succeed ... and wish they could be like you ... magazine and television adverts mean nothing to you ... have no impact upon you ... comments from others mean nothing to you ... have no impact upon you ... you stick to your guns ... you stick to your goals ... you keep your eyes on the prize ... you remind yourself of all the good reasons you are sticking to your plan ... you are strong ... focused and determined ...

When you break a bad habit, you will want to replace it with a good habit, just to make sure a bad one doesn't creep in. Drinking plenty of water is a good habit, so too is regular exercise. We've touched on this before. Think of the following also as a booster.

12. 'Exercise motivation' script

You have been thinking about exercise ... you have been talking about exercise ... and sooner or later ... you are going to make exercise a part of your life ... sooner or later ... you are going to commit to some form of exercise ... and I wonder how would it feel if you went to the gym ... or joined an exercise class ... and I wonder how would it feel if you went on long walks or for a run ... how would it feel to commit to that on a regular basis ... you know what exercise means to you ... and you know what form of exercise you want to take ... how would it feel the first time you start ... how would it feel after the first few weeks ... I don't know exactly how you will feel ... I just know that you will feel good ... and you can feel yourself committing now ... now you can feel yourself wanting to start ... now you can feel yourself doing it ... now ... not next week ... or next month ... but now ... and I don't know what you will choose ... will you choose to join a gym ... or will it be yoga classes ... will it be running or will it be walking ... I don't know what form of exercise you favour ... but you do ... you know ... and you know you want to start now ... don't you ... not next week ... or next month ... but now ... now you can see in your mind's eye ... the days ... and the times ... that work for you ... and I don't know how good it will feel for you to start exercising ... I just know that you will feel good as soon as you do start ... and ... as soon as you start ... you will be so glad that you did ... and you want to start now ... do you not ...

Eating well and exercising regularly are essential to your wellbeing. So too is sleep but poor sleep is another bad habit we can develop. Progressive muscle relaxation and ten-to-one self-hypnosis can help but if they do not, then you might just need what comes next. Even if you don't think sleep is a problem for you, you might still learn a thing or two about sleep quality if you stick with this chapter, rather than skip it.

12

A good night's sleep

Good-quality sleep is essential but also fragile and easy to disrupt. With that in mind, this chapter is all about insomnia. But here I am talking about poor sleep because of bad habits, as opposed to poor sleep because of, say, stress. It's not that this chapter can't or won't help with your stress-related insomnia, it's just that you will also need to work on that stress with everything else this book has to offer.

As mentioned, ten-to-one hypnosis and progressive muscle relaxation can both help you fall asleep, but this chapter contains a script that is a little more targeted.

Before we get to that, I want to talk about sleep hygiene. This is a term that you may or may not have heard of – all it means is doing the things that align us with getting a good night's sleep. It includes:

- No smartphones or tablets at least an hour before bed (the light from the screen inhibits the production of melatonin and keeps you in wake mode, so it's counterintuitive to sleep).
- Go to bed at the same time each night and get up at the same time each morning (and don't play around with this until your sleep is routine).
- Build a bedtime routine and keep it consistent (how you get ready for bed).
- Dim the lights and wind down at least half an hour before you go to bed.

- Restrict bedroom activities (no TV, no radio, preferably no reading; keep it sleep and sex only).
- Block out light if you need to (heavy curtains) and noise if you can (white noise apps are great).
- Splurge (you spend many hours in bed, make the bedding luxurious and comfortable if possible and keep the room cool but also comfortable (around 18–19°C/64–66°F).
- Avoid caffeine, alcohol and large meals before bedtime.

If you do these things, or as many of them as you can, you will be taking great steps towards improving insomnia before the need for any therapeutic intervention. It really is an essential part of our mental and physical health, yet statistics show that 10 to 30 per cent of people around the world are troubled by insomnia. And it affects different people in different ways.

Insomnia can be transient (lasting less than a month), short-term (lasting between one and six months), and chronic (lasting six months or more). It can be due to poor sleep hygiene, stress, jet lag and bereavement, or part of another issue, such as depression, anxiety or pain. Occasionally, the cause is unknown.

Insomnia can be experienced in a variety of ways. There are initial sleep difficulties, where you find it difficult to fall asleep; then there are intermediate sleep difficulties, where you wake up during the night and find it difficult to get back to sleep and, finally, there is early morning awakening, which means you wake up far too early and then can't get back to sleep again. Early waking is often accompanied by pessimistic thinking (let's face it, if you wake up at 4.00 a.m. knowing you won't get back to sleep again, it's hard not to have negative thoughts). The things you can stress about that prevent you from getting good-quality sleep can be many and varied, as Mark will attest.

Not so smart watch

Mark was seeing me for various things, including work stress and a relationship break-up that he really thought he should be over by now but wasn't. His sleep was suffering as a result, as was his exercise; he loved to run but hadn't felt like doing it for ages. He had a fitness watch, a recent birthday present from a friend. He thought it would get him back on track. It was one that counted steps, monitored his heart rate, prompted him to rest at various points during the day, and so on. It also monitored his sleep. And it told him that his deep sleep was barely adequate. There are three stages to sleep: light, deep and REM (rapid eye movement), and although each stage is essential and we cycle through stages, the deep and REM ones are the more restorative. Therapy went well over the weeks: his stress was under his control, and his sleep had improved dramatically but, still, his deep sleep wasn't moving into the optimal zone, and he was beginning to get anxious about it. He was also getting quite obsessed with his sleep data. Towards the end of our work together, his sleep cycle was the only thing he was worried about. It was the only thing affecting his sleep. The solution was simple. Mark stopped wearing his fitness watch to bed, had no more sleep data to analyse and obsess over and, instead, simply enjoyed his eight hours a night.*

13. 'A good night's sleep' script

I want you to know that ... each night ... as bedtime approaches ... you will feel ... more and more drowsy ... more and more tired ... more and more ready for bed ... as you go through your bedtime routine ... whatever that may be ... washing ... brushing teeth ... closing curtains ... whatever your bedtime routine may be ... you will feel more and more pleasantly tired ... as you go through your routine ... more and more ready for bed ... and you will go to bed at exactly the same time ... each and every night ... the same time ... and as soon as you put your head on your pillow ... you will feel so very pleasantly tired ... your body will relax ... very deeply ... your mind will clear ... completely ... and your body will feel ... so very heavy and tired ... heavy and tired ... comfortably sinking down ... deeper and deeper into the mattress ... deeper and deeper into that bed ... deeper and deeper into that wonderfully drowsy feeling ... and your eyes quickly close ... and you will quickly fall into a deep ... natural ... healthy sleep ... sleep comes easily to you ... naturally to you ... you fall asleep deeply and quickly ...

And ... if there are any lingering doubts about your ability to sleep ... if part of you wants to stay awake ... you will find that the harder you

---

* This is a 'standard' and while sleep requirements vary from person to person, most adults sleep between seven to nine hours per night. Anything outside of these parameters isn't very good for you.

try to stay awake ... the drowsier you will become ... the harder that part of you tries to stay awake ... the drowsier and drowsier you will become ... and you sleep all the way through the night ... you sleep all the way through until morning ... you sleep all the way through until the time you have set yourself to wake up ... in fact ... if you have set an alarm ... or a time in your mind ... you find you will wake just a few seconds before ... a few seconds before the alarm goes off ... a few seconds before the time you have set ... and you will find yourself ... pleasantly surprised ... that you have slept all the way through the night ... all the way through until just before the time you have set yourself for waking up ...

The only thing that will wake you will be an emergency ... the only thing that will rouse you from sleep ... will be something or someone that requires your urgent attention ... other than that, you sleep all the way through the night ... you sleep all the way through until the time you have set for yourself ... but if ... something should wake you ... you will return to bed ... and as soon as your head hits the pillow again ... you will feel so very pleasantly tired ... your body will relax ... very deeply ... your mind will clear ... completely ... and your body will feel ... so heavy and tired ... heavy and tired ... comfortably sinking down ... deeper and deeper into the mattress ... deeper and deeper into that wonderfully drowsy feeling ... and your eyes quickly close once again ... in fact ... if for any reason you should wake in the night with no reason to get out of bed ... you will barely even remember it ... you will hardly recall it at all ... you will barely remember even opening your eyes ... you will feel so very pleasantly tired ... your body will relax ... very deeply ... your mind will clear ... completely ... and your body will feel ... so heavy and tired ... heavy and tired ... comfortably sinking down ... deeper and deeper into the mattress ... deeper and deeper into that wonderfully drowsy feeling and your eyes quickly close once again ... and you sleep all the way through the night ... you sleep all the way through until morning ... you sleep deeply ... and soundly ... all the way through until the time you have decided to wake ...

And when you wake up on the morning ... you will awake feeling deeply refreshed ... deeply invigorated ... really appreciative of the benefits of this wonderfully restorative sleep ... and you will awake feeling calm ... and relaxed ... and ready to face the day ... very calm ... very refreshed ... and ready to face the day ...

As always, the third time is the charm. Please record the above three times over yourself or play my full recording by scanning the QR code on page 8. In the next chapter, we're going to recap and reflect on everything wellbeing related.

13

A final note on wellbeing

That's it for hypnotherapy for wellbeing (more or less). Before we move on to the subject of resilience, I just want to discuss the importance of the topics covered in this section and how crucial they are to your state of mind.

I've been in practice for a long while now and lately, over the last few years or so, I've noticed a shift in psychiatry and general practice away from a pills-first prescription and towards a focus on what healthcare practitioners call 'lifestyle factors'.

This shift is due, in part, to the recognition that despite the inordinate number of pills being dished out, episodes of anxiety and depression are still rising. So now, the same professionals are looking at three other things: nutrition, exercise regimes (or lack thereof) and sleep. 'Let's improve those things,' they say, 'possibly alongside therapy and see if that helps before considering medication as an option.'

And it's working.

Nothing will improve your mental health and wellbeing quite like healthy eating, regular exercise and good-quality sleep. Hypnotherapy helps you with those things – it can give you the motivation and it can help build that healthy lifestyle. But maintenance of that lifestyle? Well, that bit is up to you. Sadly, when problems occur, when life gets too much, when we feel like we are going over the edge, it's our healthy habits that tend to suffer first. We find we're too tired to exercise, too stressed to cook a decent meal and too tired to sleep properly. And so, as well as enhancing our wellbeing, if we are going to feel able to cope with anything life throws at us, we seriously need to enhance our resilience. Which is what Part Three of this book is all about.

But before we do, here is a final script to help you reinforce everything covered thus far.

Sowing some seeds

Tasha came to see me for a variety of issues, including social anxiety and health anxiety, which had been exacerbated by the pandemic and, especially, the lockdowns. I helped her manage these issues using a combination of REBT (more on that in the next section), hypnotherapy and positive psychology. She especially liked the gratitude exercises that I had shown her and had identified it as one of her character strengths (one that had sadly fallen into disuse). She also noted that kindness sat within her top five character strengths and that that too had lapsed.*

Tasha was also a keen gardener, albeit one without a garden. Science is very clear about exposure to the natural world: it is essential to our mental health and wellbeing. We need more of it, not less. The more we can engage with nature, the happier we feel. Gardens are great but having even a pot plant or two on a balcony or windowsill has been shown to significantly improve mood. And allotments can work wonders.

You remember at the beginning of Part 2, when I was talking about the five ways to wellbeing? Well, if you have an allotment, it turns out you tick every box. First of all, if you are running an allotment you are part of a community of like-minded individuals (so there is plenty of opportunity to connect); there is lots to do on an allotment almost all year round (so that will keep you active); they really put you back in touch with nature and the changing of the seasons (taking notice); many people start out knowing nothing and work it out as they go and pick up tips from the people around them (so you're always learning); and, finally, there is a lot of kindness and generosity in an allotment community (swapping, sharing and giving seeds, plants, vegetables, equipment and time). In

---

* If you would like to know your character strengths, you can take a free online test at www.viacharacter.org

fact, if you want to sort out your wellbeing right now, see if you can get an allotment.

Tasha tried exactly that but there was a very long waiting list. However, at the edge of the development in which she lived there was an overgrown patch of scrubland that may or may not have once been a large grass verge. No one appeared to use or maintain it. She contacted the council. They owned the land but hadn't really taken ownership of it. She asked if she could do something with it and the council said yes. She began clearing it, weeding it and then planting seeds for various plants, flowers, herbs and vegetables. Other neighbours noticed and commented. Some offered advice, others gave her plants and a few joined in. And in almost no time at all, what was once an overgrown grass verge became a community garden. More importantly, Tasha herself had followed her own intuition, with a few seeds sown in therapy, developed her own wellbeing plan and was now actively playing to two of her character strengths and tackling her anxieties head-on.

14. 'You reap what you sow' script

I want you to see ... or sense ... or imagine yourself ... standing in a beautiful garden ... tall trees line the garden, their branches gently swaying ... their leaves gently rustling softly in the breeze ... the sweet smells and aromas from a variety of bushes and plants waft gently past and catch your attention ... you savour them for a moment ... pleasantly surprised at how many you can identify ... perhaps you can see a pond in your garden ... with fish swimming in its depths ... with insects darting across its surface ... perhaps there is a rockery ... full of interesting plants and shrubs ... but what catches your eye ... is a good-sized patch of land that has been neglected ... that lies overgrown with weeds ... by the patch of weeds is a wooden shed ... and in the wooden shed ... are all the tools you need to work on and improve ... this overgrown patch of land ... and you know what to do ... you know what you want to do ... and so you dig and you weed ... you leave the weeds in a heap to one side ... there to wither and die in the sun ... you till the earth ... make it fresh ... and mix it with compost from the shed ... and then you plant a variety of seeds ... now I don't know what seeds you will find in that shed ... and I don't know what seeds you will plant ... will it be seeds that grow into fresh fruit and vegetables for you to use in your new healthy diet ... will they be the seeds of shrubs and flowers ... that require a lot of maintenance ... and mean a lot of beneficial exercise ... will there be seeds for plants such as lavender ... so aromatic ... so soporific ... something to appreciate the way Inéz appreciated her lavender bushes all those years ago ... they say rosemary is for remembrance ... and that is true ... but it is also true that lavender is for sleep ... lavender ... for a good night's sleep ... perhaps you are planting seeds for flowers that blossom with bright, happy colours ... there to lift your mood ... there to remind you of the benefits of positivity ... perhaps the patch is so large ... and the seeds so plentiful ... that you are planting seeds for all the above ... and as you plant ... you are thinking of who you would like to help you in this garden ... who would benefit from joining in with you ... perhaps someone you can share things with ... or learn from ... weeding ... turning the earth over ... mixing with compost ... planting your seeds ... take all the time you need ... and when you are done ... I want you to go over to one of the trees ... and lie in its shade ... perhaps leaning on its trunk ... and taking a nice ... long ... well-earned rest ...

And as you rest ... I want you to wonder ... and reflect ... on what wellbeing means to you ... on what connection ... means to you ... what activity and taking notice ... mean to you ... what learning and giving freely ... mean to you ... and what eating well means to you ... and what exercise means to you ... and in what form ... and what sleep means to you ... and how much ... just reflect on your habits ... and the things you want to achieve ... the things you want to improve ... the actions you want to commit to ... eating well ... exercising more ... sleeping deeper ... and longer ... connecting with others ... being present in the moment ... and learning new things ... and when you have finished your reflections ... just come around ... come back to the garden ... and resolve to wake up ... but before you awaken ... I want you to revisit that patch of land ... and notice what has already grown ... you will be so pleasantly surprised at what has already grown ... will it be the fresh fruit and vegetables ... will it be the flowers and shrubs that will need extra maintenance ... will it be the sleep-inducing lavender ... already attracting bees ... just notice what has already grown ... with strong roots ... and thick ... luxurious stems ... the lush foliage ... the pretty buds ... blossoms ... and flowers ... and just allow yourself a few moments ... to appreciate ... what has already taken hold ... so well here ... in the garden of your mind ... and now ... it is time to leave ... you can leave ... and wake up ... but wake up knowing you can return to this garden ... any time you choose ... any time you wish ... want ... or desire ... the garden of your mind ... with the seeds you have sown ... the things that have already taken root ... and the things you can't wait to see bear fruit ...

And that's it for Part Two. In the next chapter, you're going to learn all about REBT and discover why it's an excellent resilience-building tool.

PART
THREE

INCREASE YOUR RESILIENCE WITH HYPNOTHERAPY

14

REBT and resilience

This chapter is all about rational emotive behaviour therapy (REBT) and how it dovetails nicely with hypnotherapy. Not only will it stand you in good stead for the entirety of this section of the book, but it will also provide additional food for thought for, and therefore build on, everything you have read so far. Not bad, eh?

REBT was developed in the mid-1950s by a psychologist called Albert Ellis (1913–2007). It is considered the first form of cognitive behavioural therapy (CBT) ever created. Not only is it a form of psychotherapy (and, therefore, great at helping people deal with a whole host of emotional and behavioural problems) but it is also top-notch coaching methodology (used in both business and life coaching). Best of all, it's also considered a school of thought, or a philosophy for everyday life. This means that, if you adopt its principles in general, it becomes a great way of looking at life and all its challenges in a calmer, more rational and resilient way.

Like the hypnotherapist Milton Erickson, Ellis didn't think the past was necessarily the problem, nor the focal point for change. His idea was that it was not the events in life that disturb you, but what you tell yourself about those events – a view he borrowed from Stoic philosophy and, more specifically, the teachings of a Stoic philosopher called Epictetus (*c.* AD50–135). So, if you are stuck, says REBT, if you are thinking and feeling and acting in ways that you don't like but don't seem able to change or snap out of, it is not because of the thing, it is down to what you tell yourself about the thing. Change what it is that you are telling yourself and you get to change how you think, how you feel and how you act in the face of the same thing.

REBT isn't saying that when stuff happens it doesn't have an influence, because it does. When something nice happens you feel good and when something horrible happens you feel bad. But either way, that stuff is only an influence. More directly, it triggers an unconscious belief system, and it is your beliefs that are responsible for your reactions. Let's use an example to explain that all a little more. Here comes a model in four parts.

Part one

Let's say that I've got a series of work exams coming up that are important to me and could lead to a promotion. And let's say that I have a specific belief system about those exams. My mind is telling me something, and what it is telling me is this: 'I would like to pass my exams and get my promotion, but I don't have to pass my exams and get my promotion; I won't like it if I don't pass them and get that promotion; that would be a bad thing, but it wouldn't be awful, or the end of the world, or anything like that.'

Hopefully, you can see that that is quite a healthy and rational thing to be telling myself. So, I will probably sleep properly, revise well and, because I prefer to pass, be focused on success. But also, because I accept it might not happen, I can mitigate any added pressure. I might be worried, or nervous or, even, nervously excited, but I won't be anxious about those exams. I will be in a better frame of mind to do well.

Part two

So, it's the same set of exams, with the same promotional prospects, and they're still important to me. However, this time, my mind is telling me something completely different. This time, my belief system is this: 'Hell no! I absolutely must pass my exams and get my promotion. I must! I must! I must! It will be awful if I don't pass those exams and get that promotion, everything will be ruined if I don't!'

I hope you can sense that the above is a much more pressured attitude to take. I won't be worried about my exams with this belief system, I will be anxious. My sleep will be poor, my revision will be sketchy, I probably won't be able to retain much information. And so, on the day, I am going to arrive anxious, sleep-deprived and with poor recall. Those exams are not going to go so well now, are they?

All you need to take from this so far is that two different belief systems, held in the face of the same situation, will give you two very different emotional and behavioural outcomes. Let's just take the anxious me a little bit further.

Part three

So, I'm sitting my first exam. I'm telling myself: 'I absolutely must pass my exams and get that promotion, and it will be awful if I don't pass those exams and get that promotion.' I am anxious and sleep-deprived. I turn my paper over, look at the questions and then realise that, somehow, I pretty much know the answers to all of them. I'm going to feel relieved, aren't I? Relaxed and hopeful? Hurrah! But that relief is not safe, and it will probably be short-lived. Because of part four.

Part four

I'm still telling myself that: 'I must pass my exams and get my promotion and it will be awful if I don't pass those exams and get that promotion.' I was anxious about the exams but, having realised I can answer the questions, I feel relieved. However, with the belief system above, only one thing needs to go wrong and I'm right back to anxious again. I might begin to second-guess myself; my memory could falter, or I could plough through this exam and then immediately get anxious about the next one. This is just the first one, after all.

The point of the model above is the point of REBT, and it's this:

- All human beings (all of us, everywhere) are prone to emotional disturbance when we don't get what we demand we must have.
- We are prone to further emotional disturbance, even if we do get what we are demanding we must have, because we can always lose it, things can change, it can be taken away.
- It's only when you can express a preference but, at the same time, accept that you don't have to have it (even though you want it), then you can remain psychologically healthy.

● In the above, this means the difference between unhealthily anxious about the exams or healthily concerned (or nervous) about the same exams.

As easy as ...

Ellis came up with a cunning approach to life and life's problems whereby Adversities (A) trigger Beliefs (B) that cause Consequences (C). You Dispute (D) your beliefs repeatedly, leading to an Effective rational outlook (E) on that original activating event. Perhaps unsurprisingly, he called this the ABCDE model of psychological health, and I will be talking in more detail about this in the next chapter.

This model helps you to identify and challenge unhealthy thoughts that are triggering unhelpful emotions and behaviours while, at the same time, helping you to formulate and reinforce a series of more healthy thoughts that will trigger more helpful emotions and behaviours.

Many studies have shown that cognitive behavioural therapies (such as REBT, CT, ACT and CFT) work well when used in conjunction with hypnotherapy. Ellis himself, a diplomate in clinical hypnosis, noted that hypnotherapy and REBT have a lot of similarities.[*]

You can even find hypnotherapy suggestions directly based on REBT in the *Handbook of Hypnotic Suggestions and Metaphors*. Published by the American Society of Clinical Hypnosis, it's not only a go-to resource for many fledgling hypnotherapists, but also the largest collection of hypnotic suggestions ever compiled.

There are only four types of belief (B in the ABCDE model) that you need to focus on. That's right, almost all negative human reactions to things can be summed up by just four types of thought (a belief is just a specific type of thought). There will be different words and different meanings in different contexts for different people but, drop these four beliefs and replace them with their healthier equivalents and you can't help but feel calmer about things. For me, and for a vast majority of the people I have helped, REBT is the de facto language of resilience. So, let's take a closer look at those beliefs.

---

[*] Rational emotive behaviour therapy (REBT), cognitive therapy (CT), acceptance and commitment therapy (ACT) and compassion focused therapy (CFT) are all forms of cognitive behaviour therapy (CBT), with similar but different approaches.

Dogmatic demands

REBT does not like words such as 'must', 'mustn't', 'should', 'shouldn't', 'got to' and 'have to'. Collectively, they are known as dogmatic demands or just 'demands'. A demand is a rigid belief that disturbs you. That's its primary meaning. It's also the rigid expression of a desire for something. There is something you want (so you're telling yourself you must have it) or there is something you don't want (so you're telling yourself it must not be). In the model above, it is the rigid expression of the desire to pass the exams and get the promotion. It's dysfunctional for three reasons. First, it's so rigid and absolute that it's out of kilter with reality (i.e. it does not allow for the possibility of failure). Second, it doesn't make sense to say something must happen just because you would like it to happen. Third, it doesn't help you; it disturbs you and disturbed people don't behave in ways that are helpful or constructive.

NB: At this point, I want to make a distinction between a dogmatic demand and a conditional demand. Contrast 'I must pass my exams and get my promotion' with 'I must pass my exams in order to get my promotion'. The former is a dogmatic demand in that it is rigid, absolutist and will probably disturb you. The latter is conditional, in that one thing hinges upon the other: ABC must happen for XYZ to take place. No pass = no promotion. Life, people and work will place conditions upon you. Your mission, if you choose to accept it, is to not take those conditions and turn them into dogmatic demands.

Below are three more unhealthy beliefs, followed by their healthy, rational equivalents to help you flip the negative thoughts and behaviours and choose their positive, constructive counterparts.

Doing a drama

People who hold demands are more likely to awfulise or catastrophise the situation, to make mountains out of molehills and dramas out of crises. Believing something to be awful means, even if just for a moment, that you think it's the worst thing that could possibly happen, or the worst thing you can think of happening (literally, 100 per cent bad). When you blow things out of proportion like that, your reactions, similarly, will not be proportionate.

The 'I can't copes'

Some people, when they hold demands, are also at risk of exhibiting what is known as low frustration tolerance (LFT). Awful is a rating of how bad it is, but LFT is a rating of your ability to deal with it. In terms of everyday language, this is where people believe things such as 'I can't stand it' or 'I can't cope with it' or, simply, 'This is intolerable and/or unbearable'. Saying you can't cope with something is not the language of resilience.

Pejorative put-downs

People who hold demands are at risk of either putting themselves down ('I am useless', 'I am a failure'), or other people down ('You are an idiot', 'You are useless') and even things (as in 'My presentation was complete rubbish'). It's a global put-down statement of the self, others or things.

There is always a demand. If you are disturbed, if you are anxious, or angry, or depressed, if you know your reactions are out of proportion to the situation, always look for the demand, says REBT. The other three beliefs fire off in different combinations, depending on the person and the circumstances. So, someone could believe, 'I must pass my exams and get my promotion and it is awful if I don't.' Someone else could believe, 'I must pass my exams and get my promotion and I couldn't stand it if I didn't.' Yet another person could believe, 'I must pass my exams and get my promotion and I am a failure if I don't.' Others could hold a combination of some or all four unhealthy beliefs.

In any context, all four of those unhealthy beliefs have healthy, rational equivalents.

Flexible preference

With a preference, you are still saying what you would like to happen, but you are also accepting that it may not (and therefore does not have to) happen. As in, 'I would prefer to pass my exams and get my promotion, but I don't have to pass my exams and get my promotion.' This belief is true (it acknowledges your reality, that you do indeed want to pass) but also accepts that failure exists; it's much more sensible to accept that, as much as you like things to go your way, they do not have to go your way. This is a more helpful and constructive attitude.

A sense of perspective

When people hold to their preferences, they are more likely to see the badness of not getting what they want in a rational way. It's called anti-awfulising, as in 'It will be bad if I don't pass my exams and get my promotion, but it won't be awful.' In acknowledging that it is not the worst thing you can think of, you are giving yourself a sense of perspective; you are seeing things as they are, so your feelings and your reactions will be proportionate to the situation.

The 'I can copes'

Instead of low frustration tolerance, try to adopt a high frustration tolerance (HFT). Importantly, this phrase acknowledges the frustration of not getting what you want, but also recognises that you will get through it. As in, 'It will be difficult for me to deal with if I don't pass my exams and get my promotion, but I know I can stand it.' This is the language of resilience, the true expression of fortitude in the face of adversity.

Unconditional acceptance

Nothing and no one can be a 'total' anything. Failing at something does not make you a failure. This is as true of yourself as it is of others and of things. All human beings are worthwhile and fallible. This is known as unconditional acceptance, and it is a much more compassionate way of looking at everything and everyone.

REBT is a system that moves people from a dysfunctional set of beliefs and on to a more functional set of beliefs. With it, resilience comes from dropping your dogmatic demands and embracing your flexible preferences; from rejecting concepts such as 'awful' and 'catastrophic' and looking at bad events with a sense of perspective; from dropping low frustration tolerance in favour of high frustration tolerance and from rating individual aspects of the self, others and things while, at the same time, accepting yourself, others and things as worthwhile and fallible at the same time. Believe me. It works.

There will be more on how this is achieved in the next chapter, but sometimes just knowing it can be enough to effect a shift and promote a change.

Single-session Susan

Susan contacted me because she wanted help with an interpersonal difficulty, specifically an issue with her partner but also some tricky family dynamics that she wanted to handle a little better than she currently was. 'I don't know if you remember me,' she said, 'but you saw me about three years ago for work stress. You really helped me, but I could do with a refresher.'

I still had Susan's previous notes on file, so I went to review things in advance of our appointment. I was expecting to review a series of sessions but I found only one. 'That's odd,' I thought, and wondered what had happened to the notes from the rest of the sessions. It was either that, I thought, or she hadn't gelled with either myself or the therapy and so hadn't come back, but that sat at odds with what she said on the phone. When I met Susan again and explored further, it turns out there had only ever been just the one session. In that session, I had talked Susan through both REBT and hypnotherapy. I had helped her understand the ethos of REBT via a model not dissimilar to the one above and I had explained all four unhealthy beliefs and all four healthy beliefs. I had also used a hypnotherapy script very similar to the one below. And it turned out that this had been enough. Susan got everything she needed to help mitigate and manage her work stress more effectively and saw no need to come back.

This happens way more than you would think. Despite the number of sessions people think they need (or have been allocated by their insurance provider), the modal number of sessions attended by people the world over is 'one'. Research later found that this wasn't because people didn't like the therapy or the therapist (which was what had been assumed) but because they got what they needed from that one session. It really is effective, but you need to be highly motivated and present with just the one specific problem.*

I'm not saying that just this chapter (and the script on the next page) will increase your resilience and I'm not saying it won't. But if you've been steadily working your way through the book thus far, I would be really surprised if it didn't do something.

What do you desire?

'Always look for the demand,' is the main maxim in REBT. Yet, without expert help, how do you find it? You may already recognise your demands from what has been explained so far but if you are thinking and feeling and acting in ways that you don't like, always ask, 'What do

---

* In recognition of that fact, my mentor, Windy Dryden, is a pioneer of Single Session Therapy (SST) using REBT/CBT – a combination that I also sometimes use.

I desire?' A demand is the rigid expression of a desire for something. When you are disturbed, the desire to be respected becomes a demand to be respected; the desire not to fail at something becomes the demand that you must not fail at that thing; and so on. Also, your unconscious mind will probably reveal some of your desires during hypnosis because it's clever like that.

15. 'An introduction to REBT hypnotherapy' script

Just relax ... and as you relax ... perhaps your mind would like to focus on a particular problem ... or challenge ... or difficulty ... or perhaps your mind would like to focus on a whole series of problems ... and challenges ... and difficulties ... or maybe ... your mind can simply focus on your life in general ...

And as it does so ... perhaps your unconscious mind would like to reflect on ... and embrace ... and accept ... all that it has learned above ... and adopt a new philosophy ... and begin to live life according to a new philosophy ...

Nothing has to go your way ... as much as you would like it to ... there are no demands ... no musts ... or must nots ... nothing is a should ... or a should not ... got to and have to do not exist ... unless there is a condition attached ... but ... in the absence of such a condition ... you can drop your demands if you wish ... it is perfectly fine to prefer ... to like ... to wish for ... something ... while at the same time ... accepting that those things do not have to be ... it would be nice if things went the way you wanted them to go ... if people behaved the way you wanted them to behave ... but they don't have to behave that way ... and things do not have to turn out that way ... understanding this sets you free ... it takes the pressure off certain outcomes ... it allows you to think more freely and behave more constructively ...

This philosophy ... affords you a sense of perspective ... nothing is awful ... nothing is 100 per cent bad ... nothing is the end of the world ... except for the end of the world ... and nothing you have faced has been unbearable ... nothing has been intolerable ... you have withstood every single thing you said you could not stand ... and so you see problems in their true perspective ... without blowing them out of proportion ...

without magnifying their difficulty ... and so your reactions become more proportionate ... your feelings become more proportionate ... and you give yourself a sense of calm resilience ... and relaxed self-assurance ... in the face of any and all adversity ... as you realise you have withstood 100 per cent of things you said you couldn't stand ...

And you accept yourself ... as you are ... a worthwhile ... fallible human being ... making a mistake ... does not make you a mistake ... failing at something ... does not make you a failure ... you are a worthwhile ... fallible human being ... we all are ... and so you extend this philosophy ... this attitude ... out from yourself and on to others too ... other people ... are worthwhile ... fallible human beings ... also other things ... projects ... relationships ... everything ... is worthwhile ... everything is fallible ...

And so you drop your demands ... you let go of your rigid beliefs ... you stop seeing things as awful ... or unbearable ... and you stop putting yourself down ... you stop putting other people and other things down ... and at the same time ... you embrace your preferences ... and the belief that things can be bad but not awful ... that things can be difficult but bearable ... and that we are all worthwhile ... fallible ... human beings ... doing the best we can ... every day ... every day ... you are doing the best you can ... and that is enough ... is it not ...

And I don't know just how deeply these healthy beliefs will embed in your unconscious mind ... or how much they will affect you as you reflect on things after this session ... I would be surprised if they had a revolutionary effect ... an overnight effect ... on the way you think ... and feel ... and act ... but I would not be at all surprised ... if they helped you deal with some situations in a calmer and more resilient way ... helped you to see yourself ... and others ... in a healthier and more compassionate way ... either way ... I think you will be pleasantly surprised ... on occasion ... at just how cumulative this philosophy can be ... and it might be interesting for you to note ... exactly when and where those occasions are ... occasions when you take a step back ... and pause ... and view things objectively ... just noticing ... really noticing when ... this philosophy comes into play ... and sometimes ... not always ... but sometimes ... a step back ... a pause ... is all you need ... to feel more calm ... more in control ... more resilient ... in the face of adversity ...

REBT doesn't just zero in on your beliefs, it also focuses on challenging them rigorously. It's only through challenging your beliefs that you can move towards that effective rational outlook. That's what the D in the ABCDE model is all about. One of the most effective techniques in that process is given in the next chapter. Get it right, and it can work wonders.

15

Challenge your beliefs

So, REBT has a framework that we can use to work on practically any problem and overcome practically any challenge: the ABCDE model of psychological health. Let's take a closer look at it.

A: Stands for the Adversity. It is the problem, the situation, the challenge; it is the thing you are disturbing yourself about. An Adversity can be something that happened in the past, something that is happening now, or something that might happen in the future; it can be real, it can be imaginary (i.e. in your head); it can be external, it can be internal (so you can disturb yourself about your thoughts, symptoms, ailments and so on). Wherever and whenever the Adversity lies, the Beliefs about it are held in the here and now.

B: This represents your Beliefs: your demands, your dramas, your 'I can't copes' and your pejorative put-downs. REBT seeks to identify these and transmute them to preferences, perspectives, 'I can copes' and unconditional acceptances.

C: This represents your Consequences: the way you think, feel and act according to your beliefs. It includes your thoughts, feelings, behaviours, symptoms and emotions. Anxiety is a consequence of your beliefs, so too is reactive depression.

D: Disputing is the process of challenging your beliefs, of chipping away the unhealthy ones and reinforcing the healthy ones. It is not only a process but also an exercise in and of itself (and the exercise is what this chapter is all about). Bit by bit, you are effecting a shift from one way of thinking to the other. When you can feel that shift take place, you know you've arrived at...

E: Your Effective rational outlook. You now operate according to your healthy beliefs. The way you think, feel and act has changed for the better. There is still an adversity, however, so you may not exactly be over the moon. But REBT makes a distinction between an unhealthy negative emotion (the emotion controls you; your reactions are not constructive) and a healthy negative emotion (you are in control; your reactions are constructive). Instead of anxiety, there is concern; instead of depression, there is sadness.

Disputing takes the form of three questions, three challenges:

1. Is this belief true?
2. Does this belief make sense?
3. Does this belief help me?

'Is this belief true?' is the evidence-based question. It wants proof. Whether you say the belief is true or whether you say it is false, either way, you need to back your answer up with evidence.

'Does this belief make sense?' is the logical question, or the philosophy question, or the common-sense question: just because it looks like that or feels like that, does it logically follow that it is that?

'Does this belief help me?' is the most obvious. You will have a goal: increased resilience is a goal, as is getting your anxiety or your depression under control. So, you simply ask, does this belief help me achieve that goal, yes or no?

These questions are very rational and objective. They cut through the emotions to get to the heart of things. And they're so rational that they are used everywhere: maths, science, philosophy, politics, policy-making, you name it. Debating teams the world over will try to outfox their opponents with questions such as these.

To highlight how effective a strategy disputing can be, I'm going to use first a case study and then a very similar exercise borrowed from elsewhere.

Way, no way

When Oliver came to see me, he was very succinct. 'I like things to be the way I want, and always have,' he said. 'One way or another, that's caused me problems my whole life. I do get very stressed when things don't go the way I want.' And, by stressed, he meant anxious before the fact (just in case they didn't go the way he wanted), and angry after the fact (if they hadn't). And so, when we assessed the problem, his main unhealthy belief system was formulated like this:

1. Things must be the way I want them to be.
2. It is awful when things are not the way I want them to be.
3. I can't stand it when things are not the way I want them to be.
4. It's me, I am useless, a failure, when things are not the way I want them to be.

Oliver also put other people down, but this was after the fact, when things had not gone the way he wanted them to go. Before the fact, he put himself down.

The healthy beliefs were formulated like this:

1. I would prefer things to be the way I want them to be, but they don't have to be.
2. I don't like it when things are not the way I want them to be, but it is not awful.
3. I do find it difficult to deal with things when they are not the way I want them to be, but I know I can stand it.
4. It's not me, I am not useless and I'm not a failure, even when things are not the way I want them to be. I am a worthwhile, fallible human being.

We then went on to dispute and analyse all four unhealthy beliefs and all four healthy beliefs using the same three questions for each:

1. Is it true?
2. Does it make sense?
3. Does it help?

'Things must be the way I want them to be.'

1. This belief is not true. It is demanding one thing and one thing only: all the things going your way, all the time. It is impossible. There's no law to say it must be and Oliver himself could provide plenty of anecdotal evidence of things not going the way he wanted them to.

2. Oliver liked things to go his way but just because he liked them to it did not logically follow that they must. A demand and a preference (or a like, a wish, a want, a hope) do not correlate. None of us live in a world where we get what we want just by wishing it.

3. This belief did not help Oliver. He got anxious before the event (to the point of obsession, or avoidance, or constant reassurance) and angry after the fact (explosive and abusive).

'It is awful when things are not the way I want them to be.'

1. This was not true. He could think of many things worse than things not going his way (no one was ill, no one was starving, life still went on) and, sometimes, he could even evidence some good coming out of such a setback (awful, remember, operates at 100 per cent bad).

2. Oliver obviously didn't like it when things weren't going his way but just because he didn't like it, it didn't logically follow that it was awful. The two concepts, 'bad' and 'awful', do not correlate and one does not logically follow from the other.

3. Claiming it to be awful did not help. Instead, Oliver blew things out of proportion, before and after the event, and so either way, his reactions were not proportionate. He over-reacted and behaved in ways that were neither helpful nor constructive.

'I can't stand it when things are not the way I want them to be.'

1. This was not true. Oliver hadn't died when things did not go his way, nor had he exploded in a flaming ball of stress and anxiety or abandoned all hope. He was still here, still standing, still dealing with it as best he could.

2. Oliver liked things to go his way and found things not going his way 'a bit of a challenge'. But just because he found them challenging,

it didn't logically follow that he couldn't stand them. One thing ('I can't stand this') did not logically flow from the other ('this is difficult for me').

3. This belief did not help. It stripped him of his resilience and reduced his coping strategies to either avoidance and reassurance seeking (anxiety) or bullying and blaming (anger).

'It's me, I am useless, a failure, when things are not the way I want them to be.'

1. This was not true. Oliver could evidence plenty of successes, accomplishments and achievements so defining himself this way was simply not accurate.

2. It did not make sense. You can make a mistake, but it does not logically follow that you are a mistake. You can fail at something, but it does not logically follow that you are a failure. One (the failing) does not correlate with the other (being a failure).

3. It didn't help. Putting himself down was a big trigger to his insecurities and anxieties.

'I would prefer things to be the way I want them to be, but they don't have to be.'

1. This was true (Oliver felt better when things were going his way); but it was also true that they didn't have to, and he could evidence plenty of times when they hadn't.

2. When expressed this way, things make sense; it accepts the way the world works and one concept ('does not have to') logically follows from the other ('I would prefer it').

3. Oliver could see this would help. 'I would calm the fuck down,' he said, rather succinctly.

'I don't like it when things are not the way I want them to be, but it is not awful.'

1. Oliver didn't like it when things didn't go according to plan (so, for him, it was a bad thing) but it was not the worst thing he could think of happening (therefore 'not awful' was also true).

2. This belief makes sense. Things can be bad but logically, they cannot be awful. Here, one concept correlates with the other.

3. This belief gave Oliver a sense of perspective. It allowed him to react proportionately to the situation, with worry of different levels to different things but without the panic and the anxiety. Therefore, it was helpful.

'I do find it difficult to deal with when things are not the way I want them to be, but I know I can stand it.'

1. This belief was true. Oliver's current modus operandi of anxiety was evidence of the difficulty, but the fact that he was alive and anxious was proof that he was standing it, albeit with difficulty.
2. This belief was logical. Just because it is difficult, the only sensible conclusion is that he was standing it (albeit with difficulty). One concept correlated with the other.
3. This belief would help. Oliver said he would not only feel calmer and more capable with this belief but also more resilient and in control.

'I'm not useless, or a failure, even when things are not the way I want them to be. I am a worthwhile, fallible human being.'

1. This was true. First, Oliver could evidence success and achievement (so he was not useless and not a failure) but he could also evidence mistakes and failures (thus proving he was fallible). As for the worthwhile bit ... Well, loosely translated, this means 'sufficient as is' or 'sufficiently valuable or important to be worth one's time' (and so everyone is worthwhile).
2. It makes sense as one failing (or even a few failings) does not a failure make. You can rate individual aspects of the self but the only logical conclusion to that is that you are still worthwhile and fallible.
3. This belief would help. 'I would feel so much better about myself,' he said.

Momentous lightbulb moments

Some people claim that disputing is just me pointing out the bleeding obvious. 'Yes,' I agree quite happily. 'Because pointing out the bleeding obvious is not something you do in moments of disturbance.'

For others, however, it can be quite life-changing. Oliver had a revelation during the disputing process (you could almost literally see the metaphorical lightbulbs going off and brightening the room). When he came back the following week, he didn't think he needed to see me anymore. When I asked why not, he said, 'Nothing's awful, nothing's unbearable, we're all fine. I am fine as I am.'

After the disputing session, he had not only dismantled his beliefs, but he'd also pretty much dismantled his whole life and resolved to be the more rational and resilient version of himself going forwards. In fact, two work-related things had not gone his way and he took them both in his stride. 'That's great,' I said, 'but let's play it safe. Why not book a session for a month from now to see how you are doing?'

A few days before that session, I got a text from Oliver cancelling the session as he didn't need it. 'Nothing's awful,' he wrote. 'Nothing is unbearable, we're all fine. I am fine as I am.' And he included a smiley face emoji. But just to be extra safe, I offered him another safety net session in three months' time. A week before that session, he phoned me up. 'I don't need the session,' he said. 'Nothing's awful, nothing's unbearable, we're all fine. I am fine as I am.' He thanked me for what had been the most revelatory and helpful 50 minutes of his life and we brought therapy to a close.

Disputing is such an excellent tool that it's used elsewhere, including positive psychology, which considers it an essential resilience-building exercise.

Real time resilience (RTR)

This is an elegant four-step process that allows you to take a negative thought, challenge it and turn it into a more helpful, solution-focused thought. With practice, you can get so good at it that you can do it on the fly, as and when the need arises. Versions of it are used in business management resilience workshops the world over and it's so effective that it's used in US Army training. 'Real-Time Resilience is a skill that uses evidence, optimism, and putting things in perspective to fight counterproductive thoughts in the moment and takes us to a place of self-confidence,' it says on the Army Ready and Resilience website.

With RTR, you write down an unhelpful thought and challenge it immediately. You then formulate a healthy alternative and a strategy that fits that alternative ('If "X" happens, then I will do "Y".'). And so, with those four steps, what started out as a stressful thought quickly becomes a helpful thought with a solution attached to it.

For instance, this was an RTR exercise a client of mine, Andrew, came up with. Andrew had never really liked public speaking. He didn't like speaking in work meetings and he really didn't like leading them. And he hated presentations, seminars and speeches where he had to present and speak. In fact, he had avoided them as much as possible his whole working life. The problem was that he had just been promoted into a role that would involve lots of meetings, client-facing discussions, presentations, webinars and more. We used REBT and hypnotherapy to help him deal with his anxieties in this area and RTR cue cards to help him further still. This was one such card.

Andrew's RTR Card

Unhelpful thought:	I am nearing the end of my presentation, the Q&A is next, what if I get asked a question and I can't answer it, that would be terrible. I will look like such an idiot in front of everyone.
Dispute:	That's not true. Not answering a question is not terrible. I won't like it, but it's not the worst thing that could happen. And I won't look like an idiot. It's a mild embarrassment at best.
Helpful alternative:	You're right. I've seen people unable to answer questions before. Nothing ever happens. People don't think badly of them after and, while I know I don't know everything, I do know more than I think I do. I can relax. I've got this.
If 'X' then 'Y':	If someone asks me a question and I can't answer it, I will take their contact details down and promise to get back to them within 24 hours.

16. 'Disputing hypnosis session' script

As you relax ... I want you to reflect on your unhealthy beliefs ... on your demands ... on the things you believe must or must not happen ... should or should not happen ... and ... on the things you think are awful ... or a catastrophe ... or a nightmare come true ... on the things you think you cannot stand or cope with ... the situations and people you find intolerable ... the language you use to describe yourself and others ... all-defining statements such as failure ... or useless ... or worthless ... or idiot ...

Because ... you now know ... that none of these beliefs are true ... that none of these attitudes are sensible ... and that none of these thoughts are helpful to you or to others ...

Demands are not true ... because the alternative always exists and you have plenty of examples of that happening ... and you can reflect on a few of those examples now ... all the evidence you need ... and while it would be nice to live in a world where we got what we wanted just by wishing for it ... or boring ... depending on your point of view ... you know you do not live in a world where that happens ... a wish is one thing ... but a demand is another ... and you know that holding demands do not help you ... they disturb you ... they make you think ... and feel ... and act in ways that are not helpful ... are not constructive ...

And you now know ... that nothing is awful ... nothing is terrible ... nothing is the end of the world ... except for the end of the world ... you can always think of worse ... and so awful ... is simply not true ... and while something can be bad ... to some degree or other ... depending on the situation ... it does not make sense to turn that bad thing ... into an awful thing ... and it does not help you ... it makes mountains out of molehills ... it makes dramas out of crises ... and so your reactions ... are never proportionate to the situation ...

And you also know that it is not true ... to say something is unbearable ... that you cannot cope ... or stand it ... there are things in this world you cannot stand ... extreme heat can kill you ... extreme cold can kill you ... but you are standing the thing you claim you cannot stand ... you are alive ... you are the proof that it is not true ... and you know ... that difficult is one thing ... and that unbearable is another thing entirely ... and that one does not logically connect to the other ... and it does not help you to say ... you cannot stand it ... it strips away your healthy coping strategies ... it chips away at your resilience ... it allows unhealthy coping strategies to creep in ...

And you now know ... and understand ... that nothing and no one ... including yourself ... is stupid ... or a failure ... or useless in any way ... you can evidence good points ... good elements ... achievements and successes ... and you know that you can fail at something but it makes no sense to define anyone or anything by that failing ... and it doesn't help you ... it is so much easier to become upset with yourself ... and with others ... if you see either them or yourself as inferior in some way ... deficient because of an error or character flaw ...

And so ... you reject these beliefs ... you reject your demands ... you reject your awful beliefs ... your can't stand it beliefs ... and you reject your pejorative put-downs ...

Now ... I want you to reflect on your healthy beliefs ... on your flexible preferences ... on the things you want ... but accept don't have to be ... on the things you don't want to happen ... but accept there is nothing to say they must not happen ... and ... on the things you know to be bad but not awful ... nor a catastrophe ... nor a nightmare come true ... on the things you know are difficult for you to deal with ... challenging at times ... but situations and people you know you can cope with ... that you can endure ... and I want you to know ... deeply ... on an intuitive level ... that nothing and no one is ... a failure ... or useless ... or worthless ... or an idiot ... everyone is worthwhile ... everyone is fallible ... everything contains elements of both good and bad ...

Because ... you now know ... that these beliefs are true ... that these attitudes are sensible ... and these thoughts are helpful to you and to others ...

Preferences are true ... you know ... and you understand ... that as much as you would prefer something to happen ... it does not have to happen ... you know that as much as you hope something does not happen ... there is nothing to say it mustn't happen ... your life is littered with ... coloured with many examples ... that highlight how this is so ... and you can allow some of those moments to spring to mind ... just for a moment ... to confirm that this is so ... and you know that this belief makes sense ... it accepts the way the world works ... the way things are ... the way they can be ... and this level of acceptance ... helps you ... relaxes you ... allows you to think ... and feel ... and act ... in ways that are more productive ... and constructive ...

And you know that while something can be bad ... to some degree or other ... that actions can have negative consequences ... that there are things you do not like ... this is true ... it is also true that you can think of things that are worse ... more bad ... and always can ... so awful does not exist ... and while it is reasonable ... sensible to see some things ... as bad ... it is also sensible to see them as not awful ... never the worst thing that can happen ... and this belief helps you ... it gives you a sense of perspective ... you see things as they truly are ... without blowing them out of proportion ... and so your reactions are proportionate ... to the situation ... to the event ...

And you know ... and understand that while people ... and situations ... can be difficult ... challenging ... it's true ... and it is also true ... that you are up to the challenge ... that you have endured ... that you have stood 100 per cent of the things you said you could not stand ... and you know that while things can be difficult ... the only sensible ... logical conclusion is ... that you can stand them ... are standing them ... will stand them ... and always have ... and this belief helps you ... it is the language of coping ... the language of fortitude ... the language of resilience ...

And you know ... and you believe ... that people are not failures ... not idiots ... but worthwhile ... and fallible human beings ... we all are ... we are all a collection of good and bad ... right and wrong ... success and failure ... and that we are fine as we are ... sufficient as is ... and you know it is sensible ... to rate individual aspects of a person or thing ... but also sensible to accept them as worthwhile and fallible ... and these beliefs help you ... to feel better about yourself ... better about others ... better about the things you put your mind to ...

And so ... you embrace these beliefs ... you embrace your flexible preferences ... you embrace the idea that things can be bad but not awful ... difficult but bearable ... and that people ... and things ... and situations ... and projects ... can be worthwhile and fallible ... both at the same time ...

Now ... I want you to imagine that you are walking a path ... and that path comes to a fork ... and you see two paths before you ... one road takes you on the same path as the one you've been on ... destination disturbance ... destination dysfunction ... distraction ... but ... the other path ... is a new path ... the road to rationality ... the route to reason ... to resilience ... and we both know ... which path you will take ... don't we ...

Mightier than the sword

Writing things down is an important part of REBT. Writing your beliefs down and actively disputing them will enhance the hypnotherapy session and vice versa. It also gives you something to read through, reflect upon and use to your advantage in moments of challenge. And that is especially true of the exercise in the next chapter.

16

A game of consequences

So, Adversities (A) trigger Beliefs (B) that causes Consequences (C). If you Dispute (D) your beliefs rigorously, you end up with an Effective rational outlook (E) in the face of the same adversity.

Disputing as an exercise challenges your beliefs in a rational way. For Oliver, this was all he required but, for most of us, we need to dig a little deeper. We need to get a little more personal. This next exercise, which I like to call A Game of Consequences, explores the way you are thinking, feeling and acting when you hold your unhealthy beliefs and the way you could think, feel and act if you held your healthy beliefs, and it does so in an emotive, personal and detailed way. Rarely do we think about our reactions and their effects in a detailed way. Aaron hadn't, until he came to see me.

Angry Aaron

Aaron had contacted me to help him with his anger management problem. He didn't like to look stupid, especially in front of other people. I quickly identified and helped him to work on his unhealthy beliefs, which were: 'I must not look stupid in front of others'; 'It's awful when I do'; 'I can't stand it when I do'; and, 'When I do look stupid in front of others, it's because I am stupid. A complete idiot, in fact.' And these beliefs had Aaron kicking off in all settings where he felt stupid or felt he was being made to look stupid. I had already helped him to dispute those beliefs, and so Aaron knew that his unhealthy beliefs were not true, did not make sense and did not help him. They all added fuel to his angry fire. His healthy beliefs, meanwhile, were: 'I'd prefer not to look stupid in front of others, but there is no reason why I mustn't look stupid in front of others. I won't like it when I do, but it isn't awful. I might find it difficult to deal with, but I know I can stand it and I am not a stupid idiot. Even if I do look stupid in front of others, I am a worthwhile, fallible human being.' And, after disputing those beliefs with me, Aaron knew them to be true, knew that they did make sense and saw how they could help him get his anger under control. He felt pretty good after that session but sadly the feeling soon slipped away. Despite him disputing his beliefs daily, exactly as he had been taught, he still found himself getting angry in situations where he felt stupid. He was feeling frustrated with himself as well as a little disheartened by the therapy. So, he shared his frustrations with me in the very next session.

'I'm not surprised you still get angry,' I said. Which was a big surprise to Aaron. 'Just because we've disputed your beliefs, it doesn't mean you believe in what we've done yet.' I paused for a while to let that sink in. I then asked Aaron what he got from holding those beliefs.

'Well, I get angry,' he said.

'Yes,' I replied, 'that's it in a nutshell, isn't it? But deep down, how do those beliefs affect you? When do they affect you? How long have they been affecting you for? Who else do they affect? What do you do that you don't like doing because of those beliefs? What do they stop you from doing that you want to do?'

'Well,' said Aaron, 'when you put it like that, not only do I get angry, I also kick off in any and all situations where I feel stupid or feel that I am being made to look stupid. I have had huge rows with friends, work colleagues, family members, even complete strangers. I've got very verbal and very physical because of those beliefs and then felt really bad about it afterwards. I've ripped doors off hinges and punched walls. I've annoyed and embarrassed my girlfriend on many occasions. I've annoyed and embarrassed myself, too. I've got a very short fuse because of these beliefs. Sometimes no fuse at all. I can't rein it in, or shrug things off, or laugh things off, which I would very much like to do. People tread on eggshells around me. I don't blame them. I can't trust myself really.'

Aaron went on at great length, talking through all the various instances and occasions of his anger and what his anger had brought about.

'Exactly,' I said, when Aaron was finally done. 'They are driving all that and more. What do you think of those beliefs now?'

'I think they're horrible,' he said with conviction.

'Good,' I said. 'And what do you want to do to them or say to them?'

'I want them to go away. I don't want anything to do with them,' he said.

'Even better,' I replied. 'Now, let's look at your healthy beliefs. If you held them, if you believed them, if you lived your life according to them, what would be different? How would you think and feel and act? What would you do differently? Who else would benefit?'

Aaron beamed. 'Everything would change,' he said. 'Everything. I would be so much calmer. I would feel so much more in control. I'd have a very long fuse indeed. Things wouldn't get to me, things wouldn't rile me up so quickly, if at all. If I did feel stupid or felt I was being made to look stupid, I could either drop it, or talk about it, even laugh it off. I wouldn't be a powder keg of anger any more. In fact, I'd be pretty chilled. I could trust myself again. People around me would relax. My girlfriend, especially, would trust me to behave myself. Our relationship would improve. All my relationships would improve. On the rare occasions where I did kick off, it probably wouldn't be anywhere near as explosive. I wouldn't get so aggressive and confrontational. I would recover more quickly and apologise more readily. I'd be more the person I want to be. More the person that I know I am really.'

Again, Aaron went on at length, painting a full and colourful picture of what would be different when he fully endorsed and lived life according to his healthy beliefs.

'Awesome,' I said at the appropriate juncture. 'So, your healthy beliefs could help you achieve everything you just said and more. What do you think of those healthy beliefs now, what do you want to say to them?'

'I want them,' said Aaron. 'I want to grab hold of them and never let them go. I want that kind of life. I want to be that kind of person. I'm going to think like that and feel like that as much as possible going forwards.'

'Excellent,' I said. 'Well, we're going to back all that up in hypnotherapy and then, what I would like you to do over the coming week is this: write everything you just said down and keep thinking about what your unhealthy beliefs are getting you and then reject them. At the same time, I want you to think about your healthy beliefs and what they could get you and embrace them. Next week, we can talk about the results. We can discuss all the effects and changes you've noticed as a result. How does that sound?'

'Pretty damn good,' said Aaron. And he did exactly as he was asked. And, in doing so, he felt very calm and very in control. He felt quietly confident and quietly self-assured, like a great weight had finally been lifted off him.

And you, like Aaron, can explore the consequences of your unhealthy beliefs and the effective rational outlook given by your healthy beliefs using questions very similar to the ones below. Those questions are:

- What do I get when I hold these beliefs?
- How do I think, feel and act when I hold these beliefs?
- How do these beliefs affect me and where?
- Who else do these beliefs affect and how?
- What do they make me do that I don't like doing?
- What do they stop me from doing that I'd like to do?

With these questions, you will be painting two very different pictures: one of a life lived via your unhealthy beliefs (big hint: it won't look very nice) and one of a life that could be lived if you lived it according to your healthy beliefs (this will look much better). In doing so, you can't help but undermine those unhealthy beliefs and you can't help but reinforce those healthy beliefs. Like Aaron, you are going to want to outright reject one set of beliefs and at the same time reach out to and embrace the other set. When you have done that as an on-paper exercise, you can back it up with hypnotherapy.*

17. 'Painting a persuasive picture' script

Now … I don't know what your unhealthy beliefs are … not the specifics … but you do … perhaps they are in your mind … maybe you have already committed them to paper … and disputed them … and I don't know how they affect you … but you do …

You know how long they have been affecting you for and in what situations … you know how you think and feel and act as a result of your beliefs … you know what they make you do that you don't like

---

* The seeds of this hypnotherapy script were sown by my mentor, Avy Joseph, on a course I studied many years ago. His version and my version are similar, but also very different, but it would be remiss of me not to credit him here.

doing ... you know the things that you would like to do that they stop you from doing ... you know who else they affect and to what extent ... and so ... I invite you to think about all the consequences of your unhealthy beliefs ... I want you to see, or sense, or imagine ... all the different aspects of you and your life that these beliefs impact and infringe upon and then ... I want you to reject your beliefs ... reject them completely ... reject them outright ... resolve to have no more to do with them ... to give them no more of your time and energy ... tell yourself right here and right now that you will give no more emotional energy to your unhealthy beliefs ...

Similarly ... I don't know what your healthy beliefs are ... again ... not the specifics ... but you do ... maybe you've written them down ... perhaps you have disputed them ... and I don't know how they could affect you going forwards ... but you do ... you know exactly what they could change for the better ... you know how you would think and feel and act as a result of your healthy beliefs ... you know what you would stop doing ... you know what you would start doing differently and for the better ... you know who else they would affect and to what extent ... and so ... I invite you to think about all the beneficial consequences of your healthy beliefs ... the effective rational outlook that they would bring ... I want you to see ... or sense ... or imagine all the different aspects of yourself and your life that these beliefs could impact upon and affect and then ... I want you to embrace your healthy beliefs ... reach out and grab them ... convince yourself of them ... embrace that potential ... and make it actual ... pull those beliefs and their consequences deep down inside of you ... resolve to live your life accordingly ... tell yourself right here and right now that you will give ... to the best of your ability ... as much time and emotional energy to your healthy beliefs as you can ... and as often as possible ...

You have painted two pictures in your mind ... one of a life lived according to your unhealthy beliefs ... and one of a life lived according to your healthy beliefs ... see both pictures in front of you now ... perhaps on artist's easels ... maybe hanging on a wall as prints or paintings ... see both pictures ... study the unhealthy picture in detail ... what does it look like to you ... how does it feel to you ... become fully absorbed in this picture until you have fully understood its meaning ... and content ... and effect ... and then switch your attention to the healthy picture ... again ... study this picture in detail ... what does it look like to you ... how does it feel to you ... become fully absorbed in this picture ... until you have fully understood its meaning ... and content ... and effect ... and then step back ... and see both pictures ... on easels ... on walls ... and then get rid of the unhealthy picture ... hide it away ... remove it ... destroy it if you have to ... and leave only the healthy painting ... on that easel ... on that wall ... in your mind ... and keep that painting ... that drawing ... firmly in your mind ... reflect upon it ... allow it to spring to mind ... as often as needed ... over the coming days ... and weeks ... and even months ...

And ... as you do so ... I want you to know that ... as each day goes by ... you can feel a little calmer ... a little more in control ... a little more resilient ... you can feel quietly confident ... and quietly self-assured ... like a great weight has been lifted off you ...

Now ... I don't really know how much of a change you will notice over the coming week ... I don't know how much conviction you will build in your healthy beliefs or how much better you will feel because of it ... I would be very surprised if you were completely convinced ... or that you felt a total change ... but I would not be at all surprised if ... over the coming days ... you felt noticeably better ... demonstrably better ... that you sense a shift in the way you think ... and feel ... and act ...

But ... you know ... and I know ... that it really doesn't matter if you feel just a little bit better ... or a whole lot better or something in between ... in fact ... there's no real reason to even pin those changes on this specific exercise ... there is really no need to know how or why something happens ... in order to enjoy the fact that it has happened ... in fact ... whatever you feel may feel so pleasing for you ... be so enjoyable to you ... that you're probably not even going to care why it happened ... but you can ... if you wish ... resolve to continue thinking and feeling this way ...

Another thing that REBT advocates, as you will discover next, is resilience through reality checking situations as much as possible. This means sticking with what you know, rather than what you think you know.

17

Stick with what you know

A lot of our problems in life, the reactions that we have (and then wish we hadn't had) stem from all the conclusions that we jump to. Those conclusions often fly in the face of reality, don't make any sense when we think about them, and often do not help. Just think how much time and energy you could save if you didn't do that. Take Rebecca, for instance.

I was working with Rebecca on her stress and anxiety, and we were about four sessions in – she had already said several times that catastrophising was her superpower (everything to her was awful, ruinous and a disaster about to strike) – when she started one particular session with, 'You won't believe what I did.'*

She had been at work. Her boss had walked past her desk at around 10.00 a.m. or so. 'Becky,' her boss said, 'can I see you in my office at 4.00 p.m.?'

'Yes,' said Rebecca and immediately assumed the worst. 'I've done something wrong,' her anxious brain told her. 'I'm in trouble, I've made a big mistake, I'm going to be told off, I've got to fix this.' In her panic, Rebecca stopped doing what she was supposed to be doing and went looking for the mistakes she had made that she was in trouble for. She spent all day not doing her actual job and looked for the problems instead, so that she could formulate a plan and cover herself. She even asked colleagues if they knew of anything, or if everything was OK, or

---

* You won't believe how often I hear that.

what her boss might want her for. As the day passed, her anxiety grew. Her dreaded 4.00 p.m. appointment came around far too quickly for her liking, and she still hadn't discovered the problem. With an elevated heart rate, palpitations, sweats and a feeling of dread in her stomach, Rebecca knocked on her boss's door and entered her office meekly.

'Sit down,' her boss said with a smile, and then proceeded to congratulate her for all her hard work. 'I'd like to give you a promotion,' she said. 'It will involve more work and a commute to London a couple of times a month and I wanted to know your thoughts.'

Rebecca was gobsmacked. The one thing she hadn't thought of, amid all the potential disasters, was that she was being called in for: praise.

Her day, however, would have gone so much better and been so much easier if she had stuck to what she knew. And all she had known, the bare bones of it, was that her boss wanted to see her at 4.00 p.m.

As REBT therapists, we focus on a person's unhealthy beliefs and to find them, we explore their cognitions (or thoughts). As we explore, we quickly go through four layers or levels of cognition: a description, an interpretation, an inference and an evaluation.

Description

Let's say that you have come to see me in my clinic. You knock on my door and find me standing at the window with my back to you. What would you say was going on? You might say I was looking out of the window, or ignoring you, or that I haven't noticed that you are there, or that I am being deliberately rude, but you don't know any of those things. The only thing you can accurately describe is either, 'My therapist has his back to me' or 'My therapist is facing the window'. And that's it. But we never stop with what we can accurately describe.

Interpretation

We often (and very quickly) go beyond what we can accurately describe. And we do it with an interpretation, which goes beyond the immediate evidence of our eyes, but in a way that doesn't carry any emotional weight. 'My therapist is looking out of the window,' would be one such interpretation. You don't know that I am doing that (I could have my eyes closed), but that statement isn't really going to provoke an emotion. But we rarely stick with an interpretation, either.

Inference

An inference is where we start to engage our emotions. With an inference, you are going beyond the interpretation and are adding colour and judgement. Your inferences may or may not be correct, but you will have an emotional reaction to them either way. 'He is ignoring me' or 'I'm in trouble' are two such emotional inferences. But again, we rarely stop there.

Evaluation

This is your full-on conclusion, based upon not only the description, but also your interpretation and inferences. REBT beliefs are nestled within these evaluations. They live there. 'He shouldn't be so rude to me,' you might think. 'This is intolerable, I'm paying for this nonsense,' you could conclude, as well as ,'My boss wants to see me at 4.00 p.m. and I don't know why.' And so, in any given situation, unless you know the person or persons involved very, very well, you will save yourself a whole lot of bother if you simply stick to what you know. And this is what I invite you to do with all situations going forwards (and with the script below). It's short and to the point. Don't forget to repeat it three times if you are going to record it for yourself.

18. 'Sticking with what you know' script

And as you relax there ... so very deeply ... so very calmly ... I want to speak to your unconscious mind about that matter of importance ... important to you ...

From now on ... when dealing with situations ... and people ... with difficulties ... and challenges ... from now on ... you will stick only to what you know ... to the facts ... you stick to only what you can accurately describe ... and as you stick to what you can accurately describe ... you will allow that situation to unfold as it will unfold ... you will let that person react ... or not ... and you will remain calm ... and measured ... and in control ...

You no longer jump to conclusions ... you no longer try to interpret the situation ... you no longer add inferences ... or allow thoughts and feelings you cannot verify to cloud your judgement ... you no longer evaluate the situation until you have all the facts ... all the evidence ... all the information you need ... you only need to fully react ... when the person ... the situation ... the event ... reaches its conclusion ...

Until then ... you stick to what you know ... you stick with what you can accurately describe ... you no longer jump to conclusions ... and ... in doing so ... you remain calm ... and measured ... resilient and neutral ...

Just think how much easier your life would be, how much more manageable things would seem, if you just stuck to what you could truly describe in any situation: 'My boss wants to see me' (instead of 'I'm in trouble'); 'They appear to be looking in my direction' (as opposed to 'They're talking about me'); 'My partner seems withdrawn at the moment' (rather than 'They've gone off me and are going to leave me'), and so on.

Another thing we human beings do, as you will discover in the next chapter, is spend a lot of time and exhaust a lot of energy on trying to control the uncontrollable. Not only is that irrational, it's also impossible.

18

You can't control the uncontrollable

Among the many sayings of the Stoic philosopher Epictetus is this: 'Suffering arises from trying to control what is uncontrollable, or from neglecting what is within our power.' And both REBT and CBT are based, in part, on the teachings of the Stoics.

The Stoics believed that trying to control the uncontrollable sat at the core of almost all human misery. And that was 2000 years ago. Just think of all the things you're trying to control today.

A Stoic believed that only their thoughts and intentions were ever truly within their sphere of control and that everything else was ultimately uncontrollable. Nothing at all; nothing else in your life, apart from your thoughts and intentions, are ever under your control. I'll just let that sink in for a moment, and then ruin it.

As a psychotherapist, I'd argue that not even your thoughts and intentions are fully under your control as, if they were, both I and others like me would be out of a job.

Lots of people come to see me precisely because their thoughts, feelings, behaviours and emotions are out of their control, and they want strategies to help them regain it.

So, nothing in this world is ever fully under your control. Zip, zilch, *nada, rien.* But before you run off screaming into the distance as the sheer horrific realisation of that inalienable fact sinks in, I just want to bring your attention to the word 'fully', because it's important.

Yes, it is true that there are many things in life that are totally out of your control but it is also true that there are many things that are partially under your control. Things over which you have a measure of autonomy or a smidgeon of influence.

Feel free to breathe a sigh of relief and, as you do so, let me bring your attention to the work of Stephen Covey and his Circle of Concern and Circle of Influence. Covey is the author of the hugely popular *The 7 Habits of Highly Effective People* (1989). In it, he distinguishes between proactive people (who focus on what they can do and can influence) and reactive people (who put their time and energy into trying to control things that are clearly beyond their control).

His model is based upon two circles, one inside the other. The outer circle is the Circle of Concern. It includes all the things that worry you but that are pretty much out of your control (global warming, the cost of living, earthquakes and other natural phenomena, the rubbish traffic system in your town and so on). This circle will vary according to the individual, but whatever goes into your circle, these are things you have no control over. So, the idea is that you stop trying to do so. You let it go. These things are going to play out the way they will anyway, so stop worrying so much about them, stop wasting your time and energy trying to do something about them. Focus instead on the inner circle, your Circle of Influence.

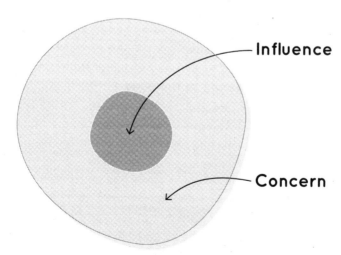

Influence

Concern

CIRCLE OF CONCERN / CIRCLE OF INFLUENCE

Smaller than the Circle of Concern, but still personal to you (and therefore variable), it contains all the things you are worried about and that you can exert some control or influence over.

Dropping one over the other gives you more time and energy, which in turn can be better spent making effective changes in key areas of your life. In addition, dropping all the stress about the stuff you have no control over does wonderful things for your resilience.

Some versions of the model contain three circles, with the third, a tiny little circle, being the Circle of Control. In it, you can put the very limited number of things that you do have full control over. But personally, I don't think there is anything in this life you do have full control over (including your thoughts) so I keep to the two circles. And while it's very easy to convey this model, it is much harder to practise, but practice is what it takes. However, Covey's circles are very REBT because they are very Stoic in nature.

'There is only one way to happiness and that is to cease worrying about things which are beyond the power of our will,' Epictetus also said.

Unhealthy demands in this area include attitudes such as: 'I must control every single situation', or 'Things must not get out of my control' and 'Things must go exactly according to plan', or 'Nothing must go wrong'. Not forgetting attendant derivative beliefs such as, 'It would be awful not to be in control of every single situation', or 'I can't stand it when things get out of my control' and 'I'm a failure when things go wrong'.

I've helped so many people over the years lead lives that were less fraught than before not only by disputing beliefs such as the above and reinforcing their healthier counterparts, but also by helping them to build their own Circle of Concern and Circle of Influence and helping them to let go of everything in the outer circle, to the best of their abilities. Not only that, but this lesson was one of the topics in my eight-week rolling hypnotherapy for stress programme that I ran at the Priory Hospital Bristol. It often proved to be illuminating (and, also, animated) for all concerned.

However, when I think of how to apply this in my own life, I don't so much think of the Stoics as I do *The Serenity Prayer*. Attributed to the American theologian Reinhold Niebuhr in 1943 and adopted by many 12-Step programmes around the world, an earlier version of it was written by Winnifred Crane Wygal in 1933. The Niebuhr version goes like this:

'God, grant me the serenity to accept the things I cannot change, courage to change the things I can, and the wisdom to know the difference'.

You don't have to use the word 'god' if you don't want to or, if you do, it can be any god (or goddess) of your choice. You could substitute 'life', 'the universe', 'spirit' or 'spirits', your 'guardian angel', your 'higher self', or anything or anyone that works for you.

But that's what Covey's circles and Epictetus' happiness represent: the serenity to accept the things beyond your control and the courage to work on the things you can influence. The ability to do so comes only with wisdom, and both REBT and hypnotherapy can help with that.

19. 'Let it go' script

Here in hypnosis ... you are in touch with ... in tune with ... your inner mind ... your unconscious mind ... the deepest part of you ... the wisest part of you ... the part of you that works tirelessly for you ... for your physical and mental health ... of your own improvement ... for your sense of balance ... and resilience ... your unconscious mind is so wise ... it knows so much ... that your conscious mind doesn't even know how much it doesn't know about what the unconscious mind knows ... and sometimes ... the conscious mind ... forgets to listen ... to that inner ... innate wisdom ... but you are listening now ... are you not ... to that still ... quiet voice ... from deep within ...

The part of you that knows ... that there are many things in this life that are outside of your control ... so many things ... that will play out exactly how they were always going to play out ... no matter what you did or did not do about them ... and some of those things ... are appearing in your mind now ... perhaps as words ... maybe as images ... or even impressions ... and here ... in hypnosis ... you resolve to let these things go ... if there is nothing that can be done ... then peace comes from you ... you let them go ... you let them play out as they were always going to play out and you focus your mind instead ...

On those things you can exert an influence over ... those things you have some measure of control over ... and some of those things ... are playing through your mind now ... perhaps as words ... maybe as images ... or as impressions ... and here ... in hypnosis ... you resolve

... you choose ... to give your time ... and your energy ... only to those things you do have some measure of control over ... only those things that you can exert an influence over ... and in doing so ... you will find ... that you will have more time ... for those things ... more energy for those things ... more headspace ... and more resilience ... for those things ...

You know ... that the only way to be happy is to cease worrying about the things beyond your control ... there is a saying ... grant me the serenity to accept the things I cannot change ... the courage to change the things I can ... and the wisdom to know the difference ... and those words are ... now ... deeply embedded within your unconscious mind ... will become activated in your daily life ... and will exert an influence over you ... and I don't know what you will do first ... will you accept the things you cannot change ... or change the things you can ... the choice is yours because ... you have the serenity to accept the things you cannot change ... you have the courage ... to change the things you can ... and you have ... the wisdom to know the difference ... the wisdom was always there ... held deep in your unconscious mind ... that deep voice of wisdom that you are now connected to ... that you can remember to listen to ... and you will listen ... will you not ...

Let it go is not only another great maxim for life, but it's also what this recording is all about. After that, we're going to tackle another big topic, namely, uncertainty.

19

Dealing with uncertainty

As well as not coping very well when things are not under our control, people often also don't deal very well with uncertainty. Which is a bit of a problem as life is a very uncertain thing indeed. Quotes about this abound.

Practically the only people who have got their heads around uncertainty are mathematicians. In his book, *A Mathematician Plays the Stock Market*, the American mathematics professor John Allen Paulos wrote that 'uncertainty is the only certainty there is,' while the French mathematician Blaise Pascal said, 'we sail within a vast sphere, ever drifting in uncertainty, driven from end to end.'

And, of course, there's that well-known saying about death and taxes.

Despite this knowledge, living without certainty is hard. We crave it as much as we crave food, sex and other dopamine-producing rewards. Studies have shown that not knowing (will I be made redundant?) is often more anxiety-provoking than knowing (I am being made redundant). Certainty helps us to feel safe, while we perceive uncertainty as a threat or danger. We then try to create as much certainty as possible to feel more comfortable.

But there is a whole world of difference between wanting to know the outcome (but accepting that you don't have to know) and demanding that you absolutely must know the outcome. Again, people who demand certainty are prone to awfulising the consequences and are not very good at tolerating the frustration of being uncertain.

How much more resilience would they have if they learned to accept the uncertainty (even though they didn't want it), made the best decisions they could with the information available, and then rode it out, accepting that while they might find it difficult to deal with, they could most definitely cope with it?

Uncertainty is a fact of life. It's another one of those uncontrollable things that people want to control. But you can decide where to put all the uncertain things in your life. Are they in your Circle of Concern or in your Circle of Influence? And you can dispute your beliefs about uncertainty. Because let's face it – with work, finances, health, relationships and, even, life in general – we never truly know what's going to happen next. We set out each morning with the best of intentions, trying to influence outcomes as best we can but, really, anything can (and often does) happen.

When you try to plan for every eventuality and second-guess every outcome it's not only a demand for control but also a demand for certainty and an intolerance to uncertainty.

It leads to an attack of the 'what ifs?' ('What if this happens?' and 'What if that doesn't happen?'). People with a fear of uncertainty often fear the result of 'What if it all goes wrong?' and rarely embrace, 'But what if it all turns out fine?'

A fear of uncertainty can lead to poor decision making, or no decision making, or constantly changing your mind. Someone must know they've made the right decision or has to know they haven't made the wrong one. Uncertainty is a hallmark symptom of obsessive compulsive disorder (OCD – often called the 'doubting disorder'). People must know that nothing bad will happen; they have got to know they haven't offended someone, that they won't be contaminated by this germ or that lurgy and so on.

To rethink your attitudes to uncertainty, try asking yourself a few insightful and revealing questions, such as, 'What would my life be like if there were no uncertainty?' and 'How would it feel if I knew exactly what was going to happen at every given juncture?' or 'What would my life be like if it held no surprises?' Chances are, your answers would contain words such as 'boring', 'dull', 'routine' and 'predictable'.

The only thing you can really do with uncertainty is to learn to live with it. Because uncertainty isn't just difficult for the people who are having trouble dealing with it, it is also problematic for the people around them. Take Lauren, for instance.

Lauren

Lauren had both an on-off relationship and an on-off engagement with her partner, Toby. The reason why it was on-off was Lauren's uncertainty. When she was with him, she wasn't sure he was the right guy for her – she questioned the relationship, picked on all his faults, made herself increasingly anxious and then brought herself to the point where she would end the relationship and the engagement. She would then make herself anxious further still, because she didn't know he wasn't the one, and wasn't sure that it wasn't the best relationship. She would then pick apart her decision to end things, regret that decision, remind herself of all his good points and then beg him to try again. This had happened three times already and she was on the brink of her fourth 'I'm not sure we are right for each other' spiral. The fiancé, aware of the signs, preempted this by telling her to get help because he would cut her out of his life entirely if she didn't make her mind up one way or the other.

In terms of REBT, her unhealthy beliefs were as follows: 'I must know that I've made the right decision for our future happiness'; 'It will be terrible if I don't make the right decision for our future happiness'; 'I couldn't stand it if I didn't make the right decision for our future happiness'; and 'I am a bad, horrible person if I don't make the right decision for our future happiness'.

Her healthy beliefs were: 'I would like to make the right decision for our future happiness, but I don't have to make the right decision for our future happiness'; 'It will be bad if I don't make the right decision for our future happiness, but it would not be awful'; 'I would find it difficult to deal with if I didn't make the right decision about our future happiness, but I know I could stand it'; and 'I'm not a bad and horrible person, even if I don't make the right decision about our future happiness, I am a worthwhile, fallible human being'.

Beliefs such as these permeated every aspect of her life, not just her romantic relationships, but also her family relationships, her friendships and work. In fact, Lauren's fear of uncertainty was so extreme and her beliefs about it were so entrenched that we spent several sessions upfront helping her to tolerate (at this point) not knowing if REBT would work for her. Technically, she understood that her healthy beliefs would help her to calm down, enjoy both the relationship and the engagement, help create a more harmonious environment and even help her to work out whether she and Toby were 'right' for each other or not. But she wasn't certain at this point. Hypnotherapy helped her to commit to the process despite the uncertainty.

20. 'Tolerating uncertainty' script

Life is never certain ... you don't have to like that ... and you probably won't ... but you can live with it ... you have been living with uncertainty your whole life ... you may not have been dealing with it as well as you would like ... but you have most definitely been dealing with it ... one way or another ...

And here ... now ... you are going to learn new ways ... to cope with uncertainty ... I doubt you will come to embrace it ... but I am certain you will accept it ... more than you currently do ... better than you currently do ...

Yes ... you like to be certain ... you like to know the outcome ... and it would be nice to know that you have absolutely made the right decision ... and know that nothing really bad will happen if you haven't ... but you don't have to know ... you don't have to be certain ... you can only do your best ... you have only ever done your best ... made the best decisions ... to the best of your ability ... with the information available to you at the time ... and that is all anyone can ever do ... make the best decision they can ... with the information available to them at the time ... and with this in mind ...

You no longer plan for every single eventuality ... you no longer make yourself anxious about all possible outcomes ... from now on ... you will take things in your stride ... be more content with the decisions that you make ...

And so ... you will become more decisive ... and I don't know which option you will choose ... will you become more of a yes person ... or more of a no person ... perhaps a balance of the two ... either way ... you will become more decisive ... because of accepting uncertainty ...

And ... if you make a bad decision ... which can happen ... if things don't turn out the way you want them to be ... which can also happen ... if life takes an unexpected turn ... because life can do that ... you can look at those consequences in a new light ... bad ... but not catastrophic

... difficult ... but bearable ... different but not the end of the world ... challenging but not overwhelming ...

You are a worthwhile ... fallible human being ... you cannot predict ... or account for every outcome or eventuality ... in accepting uncertainty ... you are also accepting yourself ... as someone who does their best ... at any given time ... no more ... no less ... and that is ... good enough ...

Dealing with uncertainty, however, doesn't just come via REBT and hypnotherapy; there are also practical steps you can take. Eleanor Roosevelt once said, 'do one thing every day that scares you.' It's good advice and a great way of increasing resilience. So, with that in mind, you could:

- Walk a different route to and from home or work.
- See a film without reading the reviews.
- Wear something new, daring and different.
- Sit in a place other than the place you normally sit.
- Order something completely different from a menu.
- Do an activity you have so far avoided.
- Try a new class, hobby or interest.
- Read a different newspaper to usual.
- Read a book outside of your usual genre.
- Talk about 'risky' subjects (politics, religion etc.).
- Sleep on a different side of the bed.
- Visit somewhere you've never been before.

The above list will require you to make some changes in your life. Important to be sure, but also quite small. However, change is something else we are not very good at dealing with, especially big changes, or when several changes come along at once. But as you will find out in the next chapter, just like uncertainty, life, especially modern life, is all about change. Before that, I am reasonably certain the script above will help.

20

Coping with constant change

We really don't like change; we're actively resistant to it in fact. We are hardwired to be. Part of our brain – the amygdala – interprets change as a threat and then kicks in our fight, flight or freeze response. This engages the sympathetic side of our nervous system and pumps us full of all those chemicals and hormones mentioned before as it does so.

Modern life means that we are constantly adjusting and readjusting to a never-ending series of changes in both our personal and professional lives. Too many changes, or too many at once, or several big changes in a row, can even trigger what is known as an adjustment disorder. Symptoms of this can include depression, crying, anxiety, insomnia, loss of appetite, difficulty concentrating or feeling overwhelmed.

An adjustment disorder is an emotional and behavioural reaction to a stressful event or change (or series of events and changes) in someone's life. The reactions are considered excessive in the face of the changes and usually occur within three months of the change. These events can include divorce or separation, a bereavement, a family move, the loss of a pet, the birth of a sibling or moving house.

I've certainly seen an increase in adjustment disorder diagnoses because of the ever-increasing pace of life mentioned above.

The famous naturalist, geologist and biologist Charles Darwin once famously never said A Very Important Thing about change. And the thing he never said was this: 'it's not the strongest of the species that survives. Not the most intelligent that survives. It is the one that is the most adaptable to change.' *

Over time, even that misquote got reduced to, 'survival of the fittest'. And since then, many have misunderstood what it meant. Because it doesn't mean strength, it means flexibility.

Not strong enough

Michael was 36 years old when he was diagnosed with an adjustment disorder and was referred to me. In a little over a year, he had moved to a new area with his wife, and then shortly afterwards separated from her. She was living in the house they had bought and he was in rented accommodation. His father had died, he had very quickly been made redundant (as a cost-cutting measure) from the job he had moved for, then got made redundant again from the next job he secured after just two months. He then found a new role that contained more responsibilities than had been discussed at interview. He found this role both confusing and overwhelming and, fearful of being made redundant again, was soon signed off work sick with stress. Although on probation, his employers were sympathetic and had been the ones to request the psychiatric assessment. 'I just have far too much to deal with,' Michael told me, 'I've had far too much to deal with for far too long and it just doesn't seem to stop. I thought I was strong, I thought I could stand up to anything, but now I just feel weak.' And that was the crux of the problem and so that is what we worked on.

There were several aspects to this that Michael wanted to work on but the unhealthy beliefs behind his main presenting issue were: 'I should be stronger than this'; 'It is awful that I am not stronger than this'; 'I can't stand it that I am not stronger than this'; and 'I am weak and a failure for not being stronger than this'.

---

* It's supposedly from *On the Origin of the Species*, only, he didn't write it. Not quite like that anyway. He did say something similar, but different. This misattribution, however, is not only all over the internet, but also etched into the stone floor of the headquarters of the American Academy of Arts and Sciences (they even had Darwin's name carved under the quotation, until they realised their error and removed it).

His healthy beliefs were: 'I would like to be stronger than this, but I don't have to be stronger than this'; 'I don't like it that I'm not stronger than this, but it isn't awful'; 'I find it difficult to deal with the fact that I am not stronger than this, but I know I can stand it'; and 'I am neither weak, nor a failure, even though I am not stronger than this, I am a worthwhile, fallible human being'.

Using both hypnotherapy and REBT (including disputing, persuasion and other exercises) and a variety of scripts not too dissimilar to the one given below, we helped move Michael from a position of unhealthy anxiety to healthy concern, from feeling overwhelmed to, simply, 'whelmed' and from feeling like he couldn't cope with all his stuff, to feeling like he could cope with it, even though there was the same amount of stuff.* He returned to work, passed his probationary period, and got both his personal and professional life back on track.

Life is change and nothing lasts forever, neither the good things, nor the bad things, and not the changes you are experiencing. We do know that but, sometimes, in the moment, when our unhealthy beliefs kick in and irrationality rules the roost, we forget that nothing lasts forever and that – good and bad; right and wrong; easy and challenging – there is always another side; one that we come out of.

21. 'This too shall pass' script

Change is inevitable ... it's true ... and it's also true ... that nothing lasts forever ... all things pass ... and when the changes are big changes ... or when they are coming on thick and fast ... I want you to know ... that you are going to get really good ... at dealing with those changes ... because you know ... deep down ... that as big as they are ... they will pass ... as many as there are ... they will pass ... and things will return to their status quo ... they always do ...

Charles Darwin ... is famous for his theory of evolution ... survival of the fittest ... but ... by fittest ... he didn't mean the strongest ... he

---

* Whelmed is a word. It used to mean 'to bury, engulf, or submerge', however, in the comedy *10 Things I Hate About You* (1999), one of the characters, Chastity Church, cried, 'I know you can be underwhelmed, and you can be overwhelmed, but can you ever just be whelmed?' And with that, a new definition was born. Since then, 'whelmed' has been used to describe a happy ground, a mid-point between over- and underwhelmed. Even language is subject to change. Some people have a harder time dealing with that than others.

meant the most adaptable ... those most able to adapt to the changes they are presented with ... to go with the flow ... even when the flow was not ideal ... and you have survived 100 per cent of the things you thought you would never get through ... and you will survive all the other changes in your life ... by being adaptable to change ... by being flexible in the face of change ... rather than rigid and resistant to change ... change is inevitable ... and you know there is no point in resisting the inevitable ... and so you go with the flow ... doing your best in challenging times ... keeping a sense of perspective ... keeping a sense of proportion ... accepting yourself as worthwhile ... but fallible ... doing your best ... as you always do ... making mistakes ... as everybody does ... there is a phrase ... a saying ... a reflection on the human condition ... an understanding that neither the good moments ... nor the bad moments ... in life ... last forever ... this too shall pass ... the saying goes ... this too shall pass ... and as you meet your challenges ... and changes ... calmly ... flexibly ... seeing things as bad ... to some degree or other ... but never the worst thing that could be ... difficult ... to some degree or other ... but never unbearably so ... and that any and all concerned in the matter ... including yourself ... are fine as they are ... doing their best ... you know ... and you understand ... and you believe ... that ... this too shall pass ... . you are fit ... you are flexible ... you are adaptable ... and this too shall pass ...

This chapter too shall pass. The next one is all about how to assert yourself more effectively.

21

Assertiveness training

Sarah came to see me because she was too meek and mild. 'I'm a bit of a pushover,' she said. Sarah didn't like to make a kerfuffle, either personally or professionally. Friends had told her that she needed to stand up for herself more. At work, she had been told a similar thing if her career was to progress any further. But she didn't like to cause a scene and upset people. This attitude formed the basis of her beliefs, which were: 'I must not upset people'; 'It would be awful if I upset people'; 'I couldn't stand it if I upset people'; and 'I am a bad person if I upset people'.

These beliefs gave Sarah a passive personality with an equally passive communication style. Passive communicators fail to assert themselves, allow people to infringe upon their rights, fail to express their feelings, needs or opinions, tend to speak softly and/or apologetically, make poor eye contact and tend to make themselves seem small when talking to others. They can often feel anxious, depressed, resentful and even confused (because they ignore their own feelings and needs).

Sarah recognised herself in much of the above and wanted to learn how to assert herself. Success was achieved with a combination of hypnotherapy, REBT and assertiveness training.

The latter started out as a technique developed by the psychiatrist Joseph Wolpe (1915–1997) who, in 1958, thought that self-assertion would be a jolly good method for reducing anxiety.

However, as a concept, self-assertion goes back even further, to a guy called Andrew Salter (1914–1996) and his book, *Conditioned Reflex Therapy*

(1949). Salter didn't use the term 'assertiveness training' but he did say that some people needed to learn how to express themselves more openly.

Assertiveness training proper began with the American psychologist Carl Rogers (1902–1987) – the founding father of humanistic or client-centred therapy). He wrote a list of 'assertive' human rights (no, not that one) called The Bill of Rights. And it has been mapped, modelled, refined, adjusted and delivered ever since. Manuel J. Smith adapted this into his own version. Known as The Bill of Assertive Rights, it is shorter, but not too dissimilar to the one listed below.

The Bill of Rights

- I have the right to ask for what I want (and recognise that other people have the right to say no).
- I have the right to have my own opinions, views and ideas and the right to express them appropriately.
- I have the right to have needs and wants (that may be different to the needs and wants of others).
- I have the right to say 'yes' and 'no' without feeling guilty.
- I have the right to have feelings and the right to express them assertively in appropriate situations.
- I have the right to change my mind.
- I have the right to say 'I don't know' and 'I don't understand'.
- I have the right to decline responsibility for other people's problems.
- I have the right to be respected.
- I have the right to make mistakes.
- I have the right to be myself (even if that is different to what others are or want me to be).
- I have the right to express my emotions appropriately.
- I have the right to have my rights respected by others.
- I have the right to choose to and choose not to exercise my rights.

Although there are many variations on The Bill of Rights, it is, in any iteration, calling for the right to be assertive. This entire book could be devoted to assertiveness training (and there are many good books out there). These are just the edited highlights.

According to REBT, unassertive people hold unhealthy beliefs around not wanting to upset others, or cause a scene, or change the nature of their relationships, cause a commotion, get in trouble, make a fuss, and so on.

Assertiveness comes through the expression of healthy beliefs about the same things. But it doesn't necessarily mean they will feel good when they do.

REBT differentiates between what it considers unhealthy negative emotions (that stem from unhealthy beliefs) and healthy negative emotions (that stem from healthy beliefs).

Some therapies say it's all anxiety, it's all bad, and we are just going to reduce those symptoms as much as possible. But REBT says that, in the face of an adversity, a negative emotion is often an appropriate response but that you can express that emotion in a constructive way or a non-constructive way.

Every unhealthy negative emotion has a healthy negative counterpart. Let's look at that a little closer. Let's look at anxiety.

Anxiety, according to REBT, is all about threat and danger. When you're anxious, you overestimate the probability of that threat occurring and you underestimate your ability to deal with it. And so, you catastrophise, you think of all the other horrible things that could go wrong. You will find it very difficult to concentrate on things. Anxious people will either avoid the thing they are anxious about (either by not being physically present, or by not being mentally present). They may tranquilise their feelings (with alcohol, drugs or food) and/or seek regular reassurance in the face of the so-called threat.

With healthy concern, or worry, there is still a threat or a danger, but you are more realistic both about the probability of it occurring and your ability to deal with it if it does. As a result, you don't catastrophise, so you can focus, concentrate and get on with things. There's no need to tranquilise your feelings or seek reassurance and you can face up to the threat (if it even occurs). You might even take constructive action to reduce the risk of said danger occurring in the first place. Basically, your mindset moves from 'It will happen, and I will not be able to deal with it', and on to, 'If it happens, I will deal with it as best I can'.

Asserting yourself, then, means dropping the anxiety-provoking beliefs and training yourself to react according to concern-provoking beliefs instead.

Sarah's healthy beliefs were: 'I hope I don't upset people, but there's nothing to say that I mustn't'; 'I won't like it if I upset people, but that won't be awful'; 'I might find it difficult to deal with if I do upset people, but I know I can stand it'; and 'I am not a bad person, even if I do upset people, I am a worthwhile, fallible human being'.

Sarah moved herself from one attitude to the other using the tools and techniques of REBT and we also reinforced that work with hypnotherapy.

22. 'From anxious to assertive' script

I want to speak to your unconscious mind about that matter of importance ... important to you ... you wish to become more assertive ... and so ... you are becoming more assertive ... you are no longer afraid to state your needs ... you know ... and understand ... that you can express your needs ... you know you have the right to ask ... but not demand ... what you want ... and recognise that other people have the right to say no ... you know you have the right to express your opinions ... views ... and ideas ... calmly ... constructively ... you no longer hold back ... there is no fear of reprisal ... you express yourself at the appropriate time ... in the appropriate fashion ... you have your own needs and wants ... and you know and understand ... that other people have their own needs ... and wants ... and that any difference ... is a difference of opinion ... there to be discussed ... reasonably ... you have the right to say yes ... or no ... depending on the situation ... and how you feel at the time ... you have a right to your feelings ... and the right to express them freely ... calmly ... without accusation ... without guilt ... or fear of reprisal ... you have the right to change your mind ... the right to stick to your guns ... but you stick to your guns with balance ... and clarity ... having listened to both sides ... yours and theirs ... and found balance in doing so ... you have the right to question ... to say that you don't know the answer ... or don't understand the question ... and you realise you are not responsible for other people's problems ... just as you realise ... that you are not responsible for how they think ... how they feel ... or how they act ... you are only responsible ... for how you think ... how you feel ... and how you act ... you have the right to be respected ... but you accept that you don't have to be respected ... you have the right to cause a commotion ... but accept that you may not always want to ... you have the right to make mistakes ... to express yourself appropriately in any and all situations ... you have the right to have your rights respected by others ... and you have the right to choose ... between exercising your rights ... and not exercising your rights ... and you make that decision ...

calmly ... and assertively ... and ... above all else ... you know you have the right to be yourself ... even if that is not what others want you to be ... or expect you to be ... and ... in exercising the right to be yourself ... you do so assertively ... with concern ... but not anxiety ... and ... I wonder what assertive will mean to you ... how will your life be different ... how assertiveness will manifest in your life ... how your behaviour will change ... how your feelings will change ... how your thoughts will change ... and how you will know ... that assertiveness is a new way of being for you ...

Now ... I want you to think of someone assertive ... someone you know ... someone you admire ... someone who stands their ground ... someone who is not afraid to state their needs ... someone who expresses themselves calmly and confidently ... and I want you to imagine floating out of your body ... and into their body ... and really experience ... what it is like to be them ... feel what they feel ... and hear what they hear ... see ... or sense ... or imagine ... what it is like to be them ...

And then imagine that you are as assertive as they are ... look at the world through the eyes of assertion ... with those ears hear the words and the sounds of assertion coming from you ... experience the tone and timbre ... feel assertion in your body ... the quality of it ... how it manifests in you ... the stance of it ... in your legs ... in your stomach ... in your chest ... and shoulders ... encode that assertion on to every nerve ... cell ... and fibre of your being ...

And ... here in hypnosis ... you know ... and understand ... and believe ... that if you ... think healthily ... act rationally ... and practise regularly ... you can become more assertive ... and as you move more towards assertion ... you will go through several stages ... initially you won't like acting in an assertive way ... and you don't have to ... it won't come easily to you ... but you resolve to continue ... and eventually it won't feel so awkward ... still not natural maybe ... but not unnatural either ... not entirely unfamiliar ... and you keep practising ... and soon ... one day ... soon ... acting assertively will come easily to you ... assertiveness will be effortless for you ... maybe you will like it ... and maybe you won't ... either way ... assertive thoughts ... feelings ... and actions ... will be second nature to you ... and that future you ... will think back to the you now ... the you now ... who is wondering ... how they will become that assertive ... looking at the future you ... who knows they are that assertive ... and soon ... you won't even be thinking about it at all ...

At the other the end of the spectrum, we have aggressive communication styles. Based on anger rather than anxiety, these people still need help in becoming assertive, but in a different way. I touched on anger briefly in Chapter 16 – both REBT and hypnotherapy are great at helping with anger management.

And that's all the time we have for resilience. If you identify your unhealthy beliefs and formulate your healthy beliefs, if you actively dispute and challenge them while, at the same time, reinforcing that work consciously (with pen and paper; with thought and deed) and then backing that up unconsciously using the power of suggestion in hypnotherapy, if you apply that knowledge and application to control (or lack thereof) to dealing with uncertainty and change and if you can calmly assert yourself in the face of any and all adversity, then you have all the resilience, all the fortitude you need to cope with any crisis, any 'thing', any adversity that life decides to place before you.*

In the final section, I want to answer some questions you might have. But before that, I want to boost your ego. The stronger your ego, the more you will be able to cope with just about anything. And hypnotherapy, as you will discover in this book's conclusion, is a great tool for strengthening and stroking the ego.

---

* Acting repeatedly, making it habitual, becoming unconsciously competent.

PART FOUR

IN WHICH
WE WRAP
THINGS UP

22

One big boost before we go

This book has hopefully reduced your stress levels and enhanced your wellbeing no end, allowing you to feel more able to cope with the challenges of life. It has helped you build better habits and improved your sleep. It has also increased your resilience by not only giving you a great philosophy for everyday life, but also tools to help in the face of uncertainty, change and loss of control. And, if you can cope with those three things, you can pretty much cope with almost anything (which is what this book has been all about). On top of that, it has helped you assert yourself in the face of difficult situations and/or people.

I hope you found this book helpful and as you move forwards into whatever crisis or calamity the world decides to throw at you next, I hope you feel more calm, more capable and, above all, more reassured. The final thing I am going to help you do is further strengthen your ego. And while I haven't exactly saved the best till last, ego strengthening is pretty much up there and is considered by most hypnotherapists to be an essential component of any hypnotherapy session.

Ego strengthening suggestions in hypnosis do exactly what they say on the tin. They are suggestions that strengthen your ego. They can be generic or specific and can increase your confidence and self-esteem. An integral part of the therapy, no matter what the presenting problem, I was taught to automatically add them to a session whenever and wherever possible.

There are many views on the ego in psychotherapy, but ego strength refers to the ability to maintain emotional stability and to cope with stress. It influences your ability to regulate difficult emotions, and defines how you tolerate change, uncertainty and frustration. A healthy ego and robust sense of self are essential to our health and happiness and to our wellbeing and resilience.

Studies indicate that ego strengthening suggestions on their own, without therapy on a specific problem, can have a positive influence on a person's mental health and wellbeing. They are considered an important part of any treatment plan.

Sometimes, in hypnotherapy, you deliver a few sessions of ego strengthening suggestions in advance of working on the actual presenting problem to empower a demotivated client enough to begin the work proper. And they are a great way to end any therapy session.

Often, when someone has finished working on the problems they brought in and are managing their lives more effectively, they like to come back on a semi-regular basis to enjoy the top-up benefits of an ego-boosting session. At other times, the ego strengthening suggestions are all a client wants.

We all live and work in challenging environments. It's easy to lose sight of who we are. The stress can pile up all too easily and can negatively affect our ego if we're not careful.

Over the years, I've helped a variety of people from a variety of backgrounds (all coming in on an infrequent but regular basis) manage themselves more effectively with such suggestions. I've enhanced both their wellbeing and resilience. The session usually involves them offloading various issues from the past few weeks or months, with me then delivering suggestions designed to keep their egos strong and stable after they leave my room and re-enter their daily lives.

I have included one such ego-strengthening script on the next page. This can be used by anyone and everyone with an interest in enhancing confidence and self-worth, or maintaining a sense of balance and equilibrium, or reinforcing their coping strategies and more.

What's more, you can use it on a regular basis to top yourself up and even attach it to other scripts in this book to make for a very full and robust self-hypnosis session.

23. 'Ego-strengthening' script

I want you to know that ... as each day goes by ... you are going to become ... more resilient ... calmer ... and clearer in your mind ... every day ... and ... you are going to ... think more clearly and calmly ... see things more clearly and calmly ... in balance ... in harmony ... so that nothing ... and no one ... will ever be able to stress you ... or disturb you ... in quite the same way again ...

As each day goes by ... you are going to find it easier to step back from your challenges and frustrations ... you are going to find it easier to remain reasonable ... rational ... resilient in the face of adversity ... and as your mind becomes calm ... so your body becomes calm ... and so you become ... more focused ... less reactive ... this newfound clarity will allow you to feel ... more relaxed within yourself ... and about yourself ... and with the world around you ... every day ... you find new ways to increase your wellbeing ... every day ... you find new ways to increase your resilience ...

And as the days ... the weeks ... and the months go by ... as you follow the advice in this book diligently ... as you practise self-hypnosis regularly ... it will be perfectly natural ... for you to cope so much better ... with anything ... with anyone ... with any situation ... any challenge ... any adversity ... that you need to handle in your personal and professional life ...

And because you are more resilient ... you will find yourself becoming more confident ... with greater faith in yourself ... and your abilities ... greater confidence through greater resilience ... greater resilience through greater wellbeing ... which will only enhance the way you think ... the way you feel ... and the way you behave ... every day ...

Every day ... you will feel more calm ... more centred ... more balanced ... even when the world about you is frustrating ... or when situations and people are not as you wish them to be ... even when things are not going your way ... you will feel a sense of control ... more able to maintain energy and equilibrium ... and at the same time ... you will feel less tense ... in the face of adversity ... you will feel worried ... but not anxious ... frustrated ... but not angry ... and so your reactions will always be ... proportionate to the situation ...

Your mind and body are relaxed ... you are at peace with yourself ... and with the world around you ... your mind is clearer ... sharper ... more focused ... and so ... you will see all problems in their true perspective ... without magnifying their difficulty ... and you will handle them easily ... efficiently ... effectively ... confidently ... without being brought down ... without becoming bothered or tired out at all ...

In the face of any and all adversity ... you will accept yourself ... you will like yourself ... you will admire yourself ... trust yourself ... and understand that you are simply doing your best ... each and every day you will value your achievements ... while accepting your limitations ... and this understanding of yourself allows you to see others in the same way too ... valuing their achievements and abilities ... while accepting their limitations and failings ...

And because all these things will happen to you a little more deeply ... a little more competently ... each and every day ... you are going to experience ... a greater feeling of wellbeing ... physical as well as mental wellbeing ... and a greater feeling of resilience ... changes are happening within you ... have been happening within you ... and will continue to happen within you ... allowing you to live your life ... in a way that is so much more calm ... satisfying ... and so much more productive ... for you ...

And that is almost it. Apart from the FAQs section (where I have aimed to anticipate and answer as many questions as I think you will pose), and then my final parting thoughts, which I hope will serve as an excellent analogy for continuing mental health, wellbeing and resilience.

23

FAQS

Is hypnotherapy safe?

Yes, it is totally safe. There are no harmful side effects whatsoever. You won't get 'stuck' in hypnosis, even when practising self-hypnosis. The worst that can happen is that you will nod off. I can and do fall asleep during my own self-hypnosis sessions. Not often, but sometimes. When I do, I either pick up from where I think I've left off or, if I have run out of time, get up and get on with my day. Not only that, but your unconscious mind is your best friend and protector. Even when you are working with a hypnotherapist, it won't let you go anywhere you are not ready to go, and it won't let you work with something you are not ready to work with. These kinds of issues though fall outside the remit of this book as we're really talking about complex mental health issues, including trauma, as opposed to matters of wellbeing and resilience.

Am I really in control though or are you just saying that?

Yes, you really are and no, I am not just saying that. As I mentioned at the beginning of this book, if you thought that hypnotherapy was a load of old codswallop and that you could not be hypnotised, you would be correct. Hypnotherapists do not hypnotise you. You already know how to go into a trance (nodding off, daydreaming, zoning out, reading a book etc.). All you do is allow the hypnotherapist to help you go into a trance, for the purposes of therapy. And you stay in that trance because you want to. You want to achieve your therapy goals. If, at any point, the hypnotherapist said, 'You want to cluck like a chicken' or 'You want to give me all of your credit card details,' you would immediately wake up and say something along the lines of, 'What the hell do you think you're playing at?' And that session would be over right there and then.

Does hypnotherapy only work on certain people?

It's true that some people are more suggestible than others but it's also true that anyone who is motivated, willing and ready to give it a go is hypnotisable to some degree or other. The more you want to achieve a specific goal, the more receptive to the suggestions you will be. As mentioned previously, we wouldn't want to or are not able to use hypnotherapy with people who are using large amounts of alcohol or drugs (either prescription or recreational), very young children, people presenting with certain mental health conditions such as schizophrenia (unless you've had specific training) or panic disorder (until that person is no longer so hypervigilant to their bodily sensations).

Aren't the people who do get hypnotised just weak-minded, though?

Not at all. In fact, the stronger the mind, the more sceptical you are upfront and the more focused you are (which is all a strong mind really is), the better your experience will be. A strong mind is an asset in any therapeutic modality. And, if you don't think you have one, hypnotherapy can help you to build one.

Is hypnotherapy a quick fix?

I wish that it was. Some people come to therapy thinking that it will be. Several people over the years have come to me thinking that I was going to 'magic' their problems away without any effort on their part. One memorable lady was outraged to learn that alongside hypnotherapy for weight control, she would also have to eat healthily and exercise regularly. She called me a charlatan for daring to suggest these things and threatened to report me to my governing body. Hypnotherapy gets you going, hypnotherapy can send you down a different path, and it can set you up for success. But you need to put that impetus into action. Whatever you come to hypnotherapy for, effort from you will be required.

Is hypnotherapy a form of psychotherapy?

The BMA considers hypnotherapy a 'valuable adjunct' to other forms of therapy, which is why you can have cognitive behavioural hypnotherapy, solution-focused hypnotherapy, positive hypnotherapy, hypno-analysis and more. Many hypnotherapists are 'eclectic' as hypnotherapy by its nature can be eclectic, so it can utilise a whole host of techniques, taken from a vast range of modalities, to help you achieve your goals.

Will I reveal all my secrets?

Nope. If that were so, you could hypnotise criminals to find out if they 'did' it or not. You will only reveal in hypnotherapy those things that are relevant to the issues you are working on and, because your unconscious mind is your protector, you will only reveal what you want to reveal when you are ready to reveal it. Whatever you wish to keep in the closet will remain in the closet. However, when working with any therapist, honesty is always the best policy. The more they know, the better equipped they will be to help you. Plus, a closet devoid of skeletons is a very clear closet indeed!

I've got very good at self-hypnosis using my smartphone, but I rarely remember the suggestions, does that mean it hasn't worked?

Don't worry, it will have had an effect. It is your conscious mind that does the listening, or the not listening, and we are not working with the conscious mind, we are working with the unconscious mind and that will remember everything that has been said to it, even if you don't consciously remember it. Some people do recall pretty much everything they are saying to themselves in their recordings, because their conscious mind was hanging on to every word; others remember bits and pieces but not the whole thing, because their conscious mind is drifting in and out of the session. For those who don't really remember anything they've just played back to themselves, it just means that their conscious mind got bored and went for a walk. Regardless of where the conscious mind is or what it is doing, your suggestions will have had an impact upon your unconscious mind.

Is hypnotherapy just the power of suggestion?

No, there is way more to it than that. The go-to tools in a hypnotherapist's toolbox are suggestions (either direct or indirect or both), as well as imagery and metaphor. Often, that is all you need to help someone. But people are more complex than that, sometimes the problems they present with are more complex than that and, occasionally, the thing they want help with is not the thing they need help with and so things can get a little complicated. And hypnotherapy has got that covered. You can regress people to pertinent times in their lives (or even their past lives, and I have used past life regression in hypnotherapy); you can float out the parts of them that are responsible for the problem or the block to healing the problem, and you can even float out strengths and resources, bolster them and give them to that part (this technique is called, a little obviously, parts therapy). You can work with people's entire timeliness (past, present, future) and on specific moments and entire sections of their history. You can help them alter or temporarily forget troublesome memories, heal their inner child (if their inner child needs healing), help with psychosexual dysfunction, enhance dreams, reduce nightmares, and much, much more. These techniques lie a little outside the scope of this book, partly because they would easily constitute an entire book in themselves and partly because some things are just better when guided by an experienced professional in an in-person professional therapy setting.

What do I do if I haven't felt the benefit of any of these exercises?

Everybody is different. Some people only need to use a script once or twice to realise an effect or put a new behaviour into motion, while for others, there needs to be more repetition, as the results are cumulative. This is a self-help book and self-help therapy books can be great, when used effectively and consistently. I have had plenty of patients who are self-confessed self-help therapy bibliophiles. They read a book, put it on the shelf, feel good for a bit, then go out and buy another self-help book when their mood dips or they slip into old ways and then they repeat that process all over again, book after book. Practical application of the things that the book suggests are essential. But if you have read this book thoroughly, listened to your or my recordings repeatedly and acted on those suggestions diligently, and have still seen little to no noticeable effects, it might be that what you need lies beyond this book. If you still place value in what hypnotherapy can provide it probably means you need to consult an experienced, professional hypnotherapist either face-to-face or online. Here in the UK, you can check out The National Hypnotherapy Society (www.nationalhypnotherapysociety .org), the British Society of Clinical Hypnosis (www.bsch.org.uk) and the Hypnotherapy Directory (www.hypnotherapy-directory.org.uk) for such a professional.*

Does science prove that hypnotherapy works?

Science never proves, it only suggests (given the current available data) and while hypnotherapy is an evidence-based practice and research strongly suggests that hypnotherapy helps with all the things mentioned in this book and more, science has yet to fully explain how it works. Theories abound and are outside the scope of this book. One model claims it as a dissociated state, another calls it a neuro-psychobiological phenomenon. Another says it's a relaxed or permissive state and one theory claims it's a form of role-play. All are relevant, but no one single theory fully explains hypnosis.

Sometimes, I can't stop smiling after a hypnotherapy session, what is that all about?

You, my friend, have experienced what is known as a 'hypnotherapy halo'. I mentioned this briefly in Chapter 2. Sometimes a hypnotherapy session

---

* Your hypnotherapist doesn't have to be local. As with most forms of therapy, hypnotherapy went online years ago and is just as effective virtually as it is in actuality.

really hits the spot. It could be that the suggestions were delivered in such a way that they carried extra resonance that day or were more in tune with your thinking or mode of speech that day. Or maybe you were just 100 per cent in the right frame of mind for it that day. Either way, you'll feel it. A hypnotherapy halo is a wonderful, euphoric feeling of positivity and joy. You will feel lighter and happier. It might come on immediately after the session (as it did for me) or a little later. It could last for a few hours or, if you're lucky, a few days.

Can hypnotherapy work with someone who is neurodivergent?

Absolutely, yes. Although the subject itself lies outside the scope of this book, people who are neurodivergent can most certainly enhance their wellbeing and resilience with the scripts it contains. Not only that, but hypnotherapy can help autistic people calm themselves when they feel frustrated or anxious, and both REBT and hypnotherapy can help them deal with rigid thought patterns. And hypnotherapy can also help people living with ADHD experience a great sense of control over their adversities, actions and thoughts.

Epilogue

At the beginning of this book, I mentioned Inéz, who had tried, unsuccessfully at first, to stop smoking with hypnotherapy. It worked for her the second time around because of her association with lavender. The bushes in her garden, their fragrance, gave her the strength and inspiration to succeed. This was important.

Because your wellbeing can be enhanced and your resilience can be increased in several ways, it can come from a variety of sources and an array of inspirations.

Words of wisdom, impactful images, meaningful stories, resonant metaphors and targeted suggestions; you name it, they all count. In fact, most forms of therapy and, especially, hypnotherapy, depend upon all these things. They are considered essential to the therapeutic process. And so, finally, as a postscript, I'm going to talk about four things that have given me inspiration and helped me endure. They won't seem connected at first, but they are. And so, I am going to talk about a broadcaster called Mavis Nicholson (1930–2022), the process of refining gold, storm-broken trees that refused to die, and a most excellent maxim for life: Mavis first.

When I was young, Mavis Nicholson presented several shows around a theme, called *Good Afternoon*, *After Noon* and *After Noon Plus*; shows that, for some reason, I have fond memories of. But before I talk about one specific memory from those shows, I would like to talk about memories in general. Because your memories aren't real and you can't trust them. Memories are malleable. They are prone to corruption and distortion. It's a bit of a kicker, I know, but it explains a lot.

Have you ever experienced an event with someone, perhaps something funny, or tragic, or odd and, years later, you are both retelling the event and yet you both have very similar but very different versions of the same situation? You both went through the same thing, at the same time and yet, here you are, telling two different versions of the same story a few years down the line. So, whose account is the true account?

The answer is, both of you and neither of you.

This is because your memories can be distorted by time, by mood, by the environment you are in, by the retelling of it and so on. Your memory is real to you, their memory is real to them and yet your memories differ. The best thing you can say about a memory is that it is today's version of an event that possibly happened that way.

This is a memory from my childhood. I was watching one of the Mavis Nicholson shows and she was interviewing an author who had escaped South Africa at the height of apartheid. Sadly, I cannot remember her name, nor the titles of the books she wrote, so I am unable to find her today but, back then, she fled to America, where she not only created a new life, but also wrote a series of very successful inspirational and life-affirming books. And hers had not been a particularly easy life.

Her childhood had been harsh but the reasons she fled South Africa were harsher still. Her husband had been murdered, her children had disappeared, and she had been raped and beaten more than once. She left with nothing. She fled in fear. But she not only rebuilt her life (new husband; new children), she built a life of love and inspiration.

'I don't know how you did it,' said Mavis. 'How did you not only deal with all that tragedy but go on to flourish elsewhere? How did you not let that break you?'

'It's about how you handle pressure,' she replied. 'South Africa is infamous, not just for apartheid but also for its diamonds. We all know what diamonds start out as, don't we? If you take an ordinary lump of coal, and you do nothing to it, it remains exactly that. An ordinary lump of coal. In fact, you can pretty much crumble it into dust in your hand. But if you take that ordinary lump of coal, and you subject it to the most enormous and unimaginable pressure then, eventually, you get a diamond. And that is how I see my life, that is how I see myself: I am a diamond in the making.'

At the time, my life wasn't amazing either, which is probably why this memory, this moment, this interview, stuck. I later learned that the idea that you get diamonds from coal is a misconception, and a common one at that.

Coal and diamonds do share a common foundation (the element, carbon). And while carbon-based life forms (mostly plants) are transformed into coal by pressure, diamonds themselves were formed millions of years ago and come from a purer form of carbon. But that doesn't matter, not to the story and not to the metaphor and, as a metaphor, you get what diamonds-from-coal is saying. For me, the message hit home, and it stayed there.

Bad things happen. Life is uncertain, the pressure often seems unimaginable. But it's not what happens to you that matters, but how you deal with it that does. Do you let yourself crumble to dust in the face of adversity, do you let it make you cold and hard as stone or do you, like the author from my childhood memory, let it make you shine bright, like a diamond? The Rihanna refrain at this point, is deliberate.

The analogy holds, even if the memory and its authenticity do not.

And, if you don't like diamonds, what about gold? To date, nearly 210,000 tonnes of this precious metal have been mined. But gold does not exist naturally in its pure form. Gold goes through many difficult processes before it can be considered pure. It has to be mined, refined, separated, smelted, moulded, electrolysed, bathed in acid, bashed about a bit, and more. I've had one goldsmith and three people who were related to goldsmiths use this process as an analogy for what they were going through in terms of their mental health. One person did it to excellent effect in a group therapy session and delivered the metaphor with such eloquence and compassion that it silenced the other members of the group as they each considered their own individual journeys and processes towards refinement.

In the face of pressure, I choose to be a diamond and, as I consider my journey in life, I reflect on the refinement of gold but, in the face of true, cut-me-down adversity, I choose to be a tree.

Nature, you see, really is the best metaphor there is. It's also essential to our mental health and wellbeing, which is why we need more of it, not less, but that's a whole other book entirely.

Not only is my story about trees an effective metaphor for resilience but it is also a memory and a much more up-to-date and reliable one at that. I even have physical evidence to back it up.

My home is an apartment that is part of a complex. The complex is built in a former churchyard. The church itself is long since gone, having been destroyed in World War II. But the churchyard is now a small park.

From my living room window, I see green grass, tall trees (maple and lime mainly), so many well-fed squirrels that we may have to stop feeding them, and several species of bird. At the time of writing, robins are nesting in a bush outside my window. I can walk my dog and watch people walking their dogs; I can observe how the light filters through throughout the day and the year; and I am calmly and contentedly in tune with the changing of the seasons as I watch each one pass into the other. I love this view. And I love the trees that are part of that view.

Sadly, several of them have been felled by the now-regular storms (climate change, another challenge, another adversity, another uncertainty). Two of them (in different years) were split in two by particularly ferocious gales. Both times, for safety's sake, the council tree surgeons came and cut them back to stumps that stood a little over waist height. Both stumps grew several branches (quite quickly) and both stumps, within a year or two, sprouted leaves from their branches and showed the world that they were still trees; shorter and stumpier for sure, but trees, nonetheless.

This for me is an excellent analogy for resilience, delivered by Mother Nature herself. You can be ripped apart by storms, chopped down by process, reduced in stature, yet still flourish. You can still be what and who you are.

One of the tree stumps was later removed entirely, reduced to woodchip and, although I was very sad to lose that stump, a new tree was planted in its stead. The other stump, however, remains, and each spring and summer, I look forward to seeing it form new buds, sprout new leaves and defiantly proclaim, 'Look at me, I'm still a tree!'

Metaphors and analogies for life lie both all around us and deep within us. Perhaps a few personal to you are springing to mind as you read this. Reminding you that you can and do endure.

It's said elsewhere in this book, but it's worth saying again: you have coped with 100 per cent of the things you thought you couldn't cope with. You would do well to remind yourself of that fact every now and then. As advice, it's worth its weight in gold, it's as precious as any jewel.

I'm not going to finish with a hypnotherapy script as, by now, I am hoping you have got good enough at self-hypnosis, at putting yourself into a trance and delivering your own suggestions, either in your head or via a recording. By now, I'm hoping you can write your own scripts and so, if it is your wish, you can wax lyrical about diamonds, gold, trees or any of your own metaphors and analogies that spring to mind. You can also reflect upon and reinforce all the advice in this book as often as you wish.

The future is uncertain, it always is. And while we can't control it or anything that comes out of it, we can control how we react to the future and all that it contains.

We can enhance our wellbeing, we can develop fortitude in the face of adversity, just as the Stoics advised thousands of years ago. I hope this book helps you to do just that.

I hope that because of it, and all the hypnotherapy scripts and therapeutic models contained within, that you now have everything you need to help you cope with almost anything life throws at you.

Finally, my favourite maxim in life is: 'This too shall pass'. Mentioned in passing in Chapter 20, it is a reflection on the ephemeral nature of life and all that it contains. The saying is Persian in origin but has been translated and used in several languages. It was one of Abraham Lincoln's favourite sayings, and he said it often. As do I. Whenever there is a challenge, whenever there is an adversity, whenever there is something that makes me think, 'Seriously? This? Now? Are you kidding me?' I remind myself simply that this too shall pass. And it reminds me of everything I have ever learned about wellbeing and resilience. In doing so, I calm down; in doing so, I remember that I too have coped very well with almost everything so far and will continue to cope with almost anything that is yet to come.

Whatever you are dealing with now, whatever you will have to deal with in the future, remember: this too shall pass.

References and resources

References

NB: References are ordered by how they appear in the text.
Accessed 2023.

1. What this book is for

'... according to the latest research, the hypnotherapy market is going to experience significant growth until at least 2030.': https://www. digitaljournal.com/pr/news/cdn-newswire/hypnotherapy-market-is-expected-to-experience-significant-growth-from-2023-to-2030-microsoft-monsanto-ibm

'One broadsheet newspaper reported that people on lengthy NHS waiting lists...': Hauschild, Dominic, 'How hypnotherapy helps soothe patients on NHS waiting lists', *The Times* (29 October 2023).

4. Self-hypnosis

'... there are a few (very broad) statistics to clear up first ... 90 per cent of all human beings can drift into a light trance': Waxman, David, *Hartland's Medical & Dental Hypnosis, Third Edition* (Bailliere Tindall, 1988), pp. 49–50.

5. A very brief history of hypnotherapy

'Braid's ideas of hypnosis...': *The Lancet* (1845).

'The first reliable example of a general anaesthetic being used for surgery was made by a doctor in Japan in 1804': Izuo, Masaru, 'Medical history:

Seishu Hanaoka and his success in breast cancer surgery under general anesthesia two hundred years ago', *National Library of Medicine* (2004).

6. Little life hacks

'However, he was referencing an even earlier treatise: the *Boke of Husbandry...*': Rolston, Dorian. 'You Can't Teach An Old Dog New Tricks (Without Learning Yourself)', *Forbes* (30 June 2023).

'Studies have also demonstrated that if you imagine a gym workout in hypnotherapy, not only will you build stronger neural pathways, but also stronger muscles': Mazini Filho, Mauro, Savoia, Rafael, Brandão Pinto de Castro, Juliana, Moreira, Osvaldo, Venturini, Gabriela, Curty, Victor and Ferreira, Maria, 'Effects of hypnotic induction on muscular strength in men with experience in resistance training', *Journal of Exercise Physiology Online* (2018).

'Musicians have 130 per cent more grey matter in the auditory cortex than the average human brain': Jäncke, Luntz, 'Music Drives Brain Plasticity', *National Library of Medicine*, F1000 Biol Rep (2009).

'Research has shown that you can improve neuroplasticity by enriching your environment...': Han, Yu, Yuan, Mei et al., 'The role of enriched environment in neural development and repair', *Frontiers in Cellular Neuroscience* (2022).

'Will Durant (1885–1981) once famously wrote, "We are what we repeatedly do. Excellence, then, is not an act, but a habit."': Durant, Will, *The Story of Philosophy* (Pocket Books 2nd ed., 2012 [1926]).

'However, according to a 2009 study published in the *European Journal of Social Psychology*, it takes anywhere from 18 to 254 days for a person to form a new habit.': Lally, P. et al., 'How are habits formed: Modelling habit formation in the real world', *European Journal of Social Psychology* (2009).

7. What is wellbeing?

'According to a Gallup study of people across 150 countries, there are five factors that shape our wellbeing: physical, financial, career, social and community.': Rath, T. and Harter, J., *Wellbeing: The five essential elements* (Gallup Press, 2010).

'... the National Wellness Institute promotes six dimensions of wellness: emotional, occupational, physical, social, intellectual and spiritual.': National Wellness Insitute. Available at: nationalwellness.org/reso urces/six-dimensions-of-wellness/

'According to the US military, it works on 96 per cent of people who give it a go...': 'The 5-step "military method" for falling asleep in minutes', *Big Think* (9 June 2023). Available at: https://bigthink.com/neuropsych/military-method-sleep/

'... one study showed that progressive muscle relaxation is also good at improving both sleep quality and anxiety in people dealing with Covid-19.': Liu, K., Chen, Y., Wu, D., Lin, R., Wang, Z. and Pan, L., 'Effects of progressive muscle relaxation on anxiety and sleep quality in patients with COVID-19', *Complementary Therapies in Clinical Practice* (2020).

'... evidence gathered in the government's 2008 *Foresight Project on Mental Capital and Wellbeing*': *Gov.uk* (22 October 2008). Available at: https://www.gov.uk/government/collections/mental-capital-and-wellbeing

8. Stress and how to handle it

'According to the World Health Organization, "stress can be defined as..."': www.who.int/news-room/questions-and-answers/item/stress

'Irritable bowel syndrome (IBS) is nearly always stress-related': Hong-Yan, Qin, Chung-Wah, Cheng, Xu-Dong, Tang and Zhao-Xiang, Bian, 'Impact of psychological stress on irritable bowel syndrome', *World Journal of Gastroenterology* (21 October 2021).

'There is a definition of stress that I borrowed from the Health and Safety Executive (HSE) many years ago...': Available at: www.hse.gov.uk/stress/

9. Stop negative thinking

'John Tierney and Roy F. Baumeister argue that it takes four positive things to overcome one negative thing...': Tierney, J. and Baumeister, R.F., *The Power of Bad: And How to Overcome It* (Penguin, 2019).

10. The power of positive psychology

'Studies show that positive affirmations do indeed improve wellbeing...': Howell, Andrew. J., 'Self-Affirmation Theory and the Science of Well-Being', *Journal of Happiness Studies* (2017).

'One such study, involving more than 1300 participants, found that gratitude exercises...': Fofonka Cunha, Lúzie, Campos Pellanda, Lucia, Tozzi Reppold, Caroline, 'Positive Psychology and Gratitude Interventions: A Randomized Clinical Trial', *Frontiers in Psychology* (21 March 2019).

'It has even been shown that a course of positive psychology for treating depression...': Hanson, K., 'Positive Psychology for Overcoming

Symptoms of Depression: A Pilot Study Exploring Efficacy of a Positive Psychology Self-Help Book versus a CBT Self-Help Book', *Behavioural and Cognitive Psychotherapy*, Vol. 47, Issue 1 (2018).

'One big study ... found that kindness positively contributes to many aspects of wellbeing...': Hui, B.P.H., Ng, J.C.K., Berzaghi, E., Cunningham-Amos, L.A. and Kogan, A., 'Rewards of kindness? A meta-analysis of the link between prosociality and well-being', *Psychological Bulletin* (2020).

12. A good night's sleep

'... statistics show that 10 to 30 per cent of people around the world are troubled by insomnia': Bhaskar, Swapna, Hemavarthy, D. and Prasad, Shankar, 'Prevalence of chronic insomnia in adult patients and its correlation with medical comorbidities', *Journal of Family Medicine and Primary Care* (2016).

14. REBT and resilience

'Research later found that this wasn't because people didn't like the therapy or the therapist...': Brown, G.S. and Jones, E.F., 'Implementation of a feedback system in a managed care environment: what are patients teaching us?', *Journal of Clinical Psychology* (2005).

'"Real-Time Resilience is a skill that uses evidence..."': *Directorate of Prevention, Resilience and Readiness*. Available at: www.armyresilience.army.mil/ard/R2/Real-Time-Resilience.html

18. You can't control the uncontrollable

'Attributed to the American theologian Reinhold Niebuhr in 1943...': Available at: people.howstuffworks.com/serenity-prayer.htm

19. Dealing with uncertainty

'French mathematician Blaise Pascal said, "we sail within a vast sphere, ever drifting in uncertainty, driven from end to end."': www.brainyquote.com/quotes/blaise_pascal_138831

21. Assertiveness training

'Manuel J. Smith adapted this into his own version. Known as The Bill of Assertive Rights...': Smith, Manuel J., *When I Say No, I Feel Guilty* (Bantam USA, 1975).

'Studies suggest that ego strengthening suggestions on their own...': Yeates, L.B., 'Hartland's legacy (II): The ego-strengthening monologue',

Australian Journal of Clinical Hypnotherapy and Hypnosis, 36(1) (2014), pp. 19–36.

22. One big boost before we go

'Studies indicate that ego strengthening suggestions...': McNeal. S., 'Hypnotic Ego Strengthening: Where We've Been and the Road Ahead', *American Journal of Clinical Hypnosis* (2020).

Books cited

A Mathematician Plays the Stock Market, John Allen Paulos (Allen Lane, 2003)

Allen Carr's Easy Way to Stop Smoking, Allen Carr (Penguin, 1985)

Conditioned Reflex Therapy, Andrew Salter (1949)

Handbook of Hypnotic Suggestions and Metaphors, D. Corydon Hammond (Ed.) (WW Norton & Co, 1990)

Hypnosis in the Relief of Pain, Ernest R. Hildgard and Josephine R. Hildgard (Brunner/Mazel, 1975)

Psycho-Cybernetics, Maxwell Maltz (Simon & Schuster, 1960)

The 7 Habits of Highly Effective People, Stephen R. Covey (Free Press, 1989)

The Dynamics of Life Skills Coaching, Paul R. Curtiss and Phillip W. Warren (The University of Wisconsin, 1973)

The Power of Bad, John Tierney and Roy F. Baumeister (Penguin, 2019)

Also by the author

The Four Thoughts that F*** You Up ... and How to Fix Them, Daniel Fryer (Vermillion, 2019)

Finding a hypnotherapist

British Society of Clinical Hypnosis (www.bsch.org.uk)

Hypnotherapy Directory (www.hypnotherapy-directory.org.uk)

The National Hypnotherapy Society (www.nationalhypnotherapysociety .org)

Acknowledgements

My thanks go out to Lara, always and forever. The dedication at the front of this book is to her. She was my dog and my best friend. I consider dogs to be essential to my mental health and wellbeing. A Staffordshire bull terrier, she was a rescue from Battersea Dogs and Cats Home and was with me for eight glorious years. She worked with me in a variety of settings. I even accidentally turned her into a semi-famous therapy dog who appeared in various newspaper and magazine articles. She died in June 2022. It put quite a dampener on the year if I'm honest.

In April 2023, as I neared the completion of the first draft of this manuscript, I met Nuala. She is an American Bulldog, also from Battersea Dogs and Cats Home and, at seven months old, she's not only a bit of a handful but also a source of great joy. I'd like to thank her for keeping me on my toes as my manuscript deadline approached. I'd also like to say a massive thank you to Poggy for her constant support. Without her, I doubt there would have been a first therapy book, let alone a second. She truly has had the best ideas and still does.

A massive thank you also goes out to my agent Robert Gwynn Palmer as, without him, there wouldn't have been any books at all. Another massive thank you goes out to Charlotte Croft, my editor at Bloomsbury, who like me, saw the resurgent interest in hypnotherapy. Thank you to Megan Jones at Bloomsbury, not only for your top-notch steerage and editing skills, but also for sorting out the referencing. I do not like styling references. Not one little bit. Thank you also to Lucy Doncaster and her incomparable copy-editing. My thanks also go out to Sam Dyson over at the Bristol Voiceover Studio (not only for his top-notch sound engineering skills but, also, for all the chocolate Hobnobs). I also doff my cap to Kate Inskip for her meticulous indexing.

I couldn't go without also saying thank you to hypnotherapist Roger P. Allen, the guys over at Mike Mandell Hypnosis and at Uncommon Knowledge. I read your stuff avidly, especially in the early days, and am certain echoes of your teachings found their way onto these pages. And I can't go without saying thank you to all those who taught me at the London College of Clinical Hypnosis as you all set me up for everything else. And finally, a big thank you to Avy Joseph, who dangled that introductory course in hypnotherapy in front of me like a big, juicy carrot all those years ago and who taught me not only hypnotherapy, but also REBT and how to weave it into hypnotherapy and vice versa.

Index

Bold indicates self-hypnosis scripts